# LETTERS to a YOUNG PHARMACIST

## Sage Advice on Life & Career from Extraordinary Pharmacists

**Susan A. Cantrell, BS Pharm, CAE**
Senior Vice President and Managing Director,
    DIA Americas
Drug Information Association
Washington, DC

**Sara J. White, MS, FASHP**
Formerly Director of Pharmacy
Stanford University Hospital and Clinics
Past President, American Society of
    Health-System Pharmacists
Palo Alto, California

**Bruce E. Scott, MS, FASHP**
Past President, Accredo Infusion Services,
    Medco Health Solutions
Past President, American Society of
    Health-System Pharmacists
Eden Prairie, Minnesota

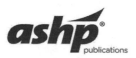

*ashp*®
publications

Any correspondence regarding this publication should be sent to the publisher, American Society of Health-System Pharmacists, 4500 East-West Highway, Suite 900, Bethesda, MD 20814, attention: Special Publishing.

The information presented herein reflects the opinions of the contributors and advisors. It should not be interpreted as an official policy of ASHP or as an endorsement of any product.

Because of ongoing research and improvements in technology, the information and its applications contained in this text are constantly evolving and are subject to the professional judgment and interpretation of the practitioner due to the uniqueness of a clinical situation. The editors and ASHP have made reasonable efforts to ensure the accuracy and appropriateness of the information presented in this document. However, any user of this information is advised that the editors and ASHP are not responsible for the continued currency of the information, for any errors or omissions, and/or for any consequences arising from the use of the information in the document in any and all practice settings. Any reader of this document is cautioned that ASHP makes no representation, guarantee, or warranty, express or implied, as to the accuracy and appropriateness of the information contained in this document and specifically disclaims any liability to any party for the accuracy and/or completeness of the material or for any damages arising out of the use or non-use of any of the information contained in this document.

*Director, Special Publishing*: Jack Bruggeman
*Acquisitions Editor*: Jack Bruggeman
*Editorial Project Manager*: Ruth Bloom
*Production Manager*: Johnna Hershey
*Cover*: David Wade
*Page Design*: Carol Barrer

Library of Congress Cataloging-in-Publication Data
 Cantrell, Susan A., compiler.
Letters to a young pharmacist : sage advice on life & career from extraordinary pharmacists / Susan A. Cantrell, Sara J. White, Bruce E. Scott.
  p. ; cm.
 ISBN 978-1-58528-399-6
 I. White, Sara J., 1945- compiler. II. Scott, Bruce E., compiler. III. American Society of Health-System Pharmacists, issuing body. IV. Title.
 [DNLM: 1. Pharmacists–United States–Collected Correspondence. 2. Career Choice–United States–Collected Correspondence. 3. Job Satisfaction–United States–Collected Correspondence. 4. Leadership–United States–Collected Correspondence. QV 21]
 RS122.5
 615.1023–dc23
                          2014005723

ISBN: 978-1-58528-399-6                    10 9 8 7 6 5 4

# Dedication

This book is dedicated to those who selflessly give of their time serving as teachers, preceptors, residency directors, and mentors for the future leaders of our profession.

# Acknowledgments

We are indebted to our many colleagues who contributed their time, life stories, and wisdom to this book. Our sincere appreciation also goes out to Jack Bruggeman, Ruth Bloom, and their colleagues in ASHP's Special Publishing Division for their vision, hard work, guidance, and patience throughout the development of this book.

# Contents

# Foreword

## Paul W. Abramowitz

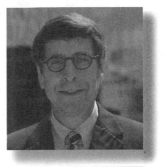

Dear Young Pharmacist,

I am writing to encourage you, as a new practitioner and an aspiring leader, to provide the best patient care that you can, to be innovative and work to improve our nation's health care system, and to give back to your profession.

Pharmacists have and will continue to affect in positive ways our nation's health care system and lead from many types of positions and in many practice settings. You, too, can seize the opportunity to become a leader in many different areas of pharmacy practice. You can be a clinical leader—treating individual patients—or you can lead by improving the health of populations. You can also lead by designing and managing care programs, directing pharmacy services, or by working with professional health care associations. Some of you will lead by educating pharmacy students and residents. How you choose to lead is up to you and will depend on your unique talents, ambitions, and desires.

Whichever path you take toward excellence, I suggest that you keep several things in mind. Continue to develop and maintain your therapeutic and patient care knowledge. This dedication to self-improvement will serve as the foundation of not only your patient care abilities, but also will enhance your credibility in any leadership role you pursue. Today, pharmacists are an essential part of every health care team and are recognized as drug therapy experts. Your mission is to get and keep your patients as healthy as possible, and it is your therapeutic knowledge that allows you to do so. Add your creativity to design new therapies and care systems and the problem-solving skills developed during your education and training, and you will be amazed at what you can achieve.

Focus on developing and nurturing relationships, not only with your patients, but also with your colleagues in pharmacy and other health care professions. The importance and value of relationships took me many years to fully understand. You can take advantage of my experience and embrace this principle early. Caring professional relationships are an essential ingredient of leadership. Make it a priority to get to know the colleagues with whom you spend a large portion of your professional life. Developing productive partnerships by capitalizing on strengths and commonality of purpose are two critical parts of building relationships. Take the time to understand the culture of your organization, and learn how to work within that culture. If necessary, learn how to change that culture at an acceptable pace. Never underestimate the value of relationships as well as the power of teamwork and collective wisdom.

Seek and take advantage of opportunities. The future of our profession depends on your willingness to exert yourself in achieving your full potential. This will take your astute observation, keen insight, and also perseverance. Some people look at others who have excelled professionally and say that they were lucky—they just happened to be in the right place at the right time; or they were lucky that an opportunity existed at that time. However, I have learned that opportunities are constantly present and they exist everywhere. Some of us see these opportunities, and some of us do not. Some of us allow these opportunities to pass us by because we feel we are too busy or we are hesitant to act on them. Some of us make an initial effort, but then retreat too quickly. However, some of you will identify and take those opportunities. Be observant and creative, and put in the extra effort. Pharmacists who excel and pharmacists who identify existing opportunities and take a risk in pursuing them will be more productive. As legendary golfer Gary Player once said, "The more you practice, the luckier you get."

Finally, I would encourage you to become involved in your professional societies—the one(s) that best meet your needs. I guarantee you that whatever you contribute as a member to those societies will be returned to you tenfold through the knowledge and experience gained and the relationships that you develop. I have found this to be the case with my membership in the American Society of Health-System Pharmacists, which began when I was just a resident. Being involved in our professional society has proved to be invaluable to me and to thousands of other members throughout our careers.

Remember, success is never achieved without challenges and setbacks. How you meet these challenges and the decisions you make to do what is right and good will determine how successful you will be and how you will be seen by your colleagues and by your patients. Stay committed to excellence, and you will find your own unique way to contribute to your profession and beyond.

I wish you the best in all of your future endeavors!

Sincerely,
*Paul W. Abramowitz, PharmD, ScD (Hon), FASHP*
Chief Executive Officer
American Society of Health-System Pharmacists

# Preface

S urprising as it seems, most professionals entering the workforce now expect to stay in a job less than three years. That means some can expect to have as many as 15 to 20 jobs over the course of your working life. It is hard to fathom, and when you think about it in those terms, managing your career seems like a full-time job. That should not concern you, though, considering all the education and training you have under your belt, right?

There is no question that the years spent in pharmacy school and postgraduate training prepared you well for pharmacy practice; however, most of us received very little, if any, formal training on how to manage our careers. How do you anticipate the many challenges you might face in your career and prepare yourself to deal with those? How can you achieve the right balance between your professional and personal lives without compromising one or both? And, most importantly, how can you avoid making the wrong decisions when presented with new opportunities or difficult obstacles?

We hope this book, a compilation of letters from pharmacists who collectively offer over 1,000 years of experience on the career journey, will help you answer some of those tough questions. These very personal and heartfelt letters address life and career challenges, sources of inspiration, conflicts between personal and professional priorities, and opportunities for enhancing professional fulfillment throughout the course of one's career.

In deciding to write this book, we reflected on our own careers, the many challenges we faced, and what we learned. We recalled situations where we might have made a different decision or taken a different path had we known at the time what we came to know some years later. It is no surprise that many of our contributors had similar stories to tell. If just one of these stories inspires you, gives you courage, or guides you in making a right career decision, we will have achieved our goal in writing this book.

With so many accomplished individuals in the ranks of our profession, selecting the individuals to contribute letters was not an easy task. We pooled our collective networks of colleagues to identify possible contributors, taking into account the evolution and complexity of health care delivery and pharmacy practice. We attempted to include pharmacists who represent a variety of career paths. Common among all the contributors are their commitment to investing in the pharmacy leaders of the future and their willingness to share their professional and personal challenges in the spirit of helping others. When we contacted them, each contributor immediately embraced the concept of the book and eagerly agreed to share his or her experiences.

It became clear early on that each contributor could have likely written an entire book about his or her unique experiences, but we had to limit each letter to just a few pages. So, after reading these contributions, we encourage you to seek out individuals and mentors in your sphere of professional practice and talk to them about their valuable experiences. Through these readings and talks with others, we hope that you will benefit from this wealth of experience.

Many of the letters incorporate the concept of leadership and its importance in achieving satisfaction in life and career. We often think of leadership in the context of managerial authority and define leaders as those individuals with executive titles, such as Chief Pharmacy Officer, Director of Pharmacy, and others. However, leadership is much broader than just the authority or responsibility conferred by a management position or a job title. Leadership, with a small "l", refers to taking responsibility for achievement of a goal or an intended outcome. It most often involves using your influence to maximize the contributions of others toward achieving the goal. As you see leadership mentioned in this book, keep in mind that every pharmacist is in a leadership role, regardless of his or her job title and number of direct reports, and we should all aspire to demonstrate leadership both in our professional and personal endeavors.

Our hope is that this book will help inspire and challenge readers to achieve their own personal and professional goals, with insight from those who have traveled before them to help guide their paths. We hope what you learn about the challenges, obstacles, and setbacks this esteemed group of contributors faced as they navigated their careers will help you better overcome those that may come your way.

What we have learned from the contributors' letters and our conversations with them will stay with us. We are pleased to be able to share it with you.

*Susan Cantrell*
*Sara White*
*Bruce Scott*

*February 2014*

# *Letters*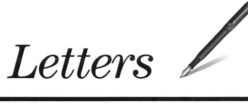

# Stephen J. Allen

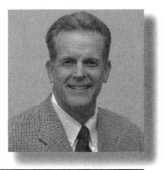

## *Give to Others, and You Will Receive Tenfold in Return*

It takes only a brief conversation with Steve for one to discover his passion for the pharmacy profession and for patient care. Steve has translated his passion into action, leading the development of many notable American Society of Health-System Pharmacists (ASHP) Foundation programs and resources. The ASHP Research and Education Foundation is the philanthropic arm of ASHP and its mission is to improve the health and well-being of patients in health systems through appropriate, safe, and effective medication use.

Steve is currently the Chief Executive Officer and Executive Vice President of the ASHP Research and Education Foundation. He received his bachelor of science degree in pharmacy from the University of Rhode Island and a master's degree in hospital pharmacy from the University of Maryland. Steve completed a residency in hospital pharmacy practice at University of Maryland. He is a fellow of the American Society of Health-System Pharmacists.

Steve's advice to young pharmacists is: *keep in mind that whatever you invest in this profession of pharmacy, it will likely return to you in tenfold benefits.*

Dear Young Pharmacist,

What a great choice you have made! It has been more than 40 years since I made the decision to select pharmacy as my profession, and I can unequivocally say it was the best

1

decision of my life. You must invest in your profession to reap the rewards, and my letter will speak to your investment in pharmacy and the personal payback that will come with it.

It is essential to me to have balance and connection between my personal and professional life. I was blessed to have a wonderfully loving family who instilled great values in me. My grandmother was particularly influential in my life. She was a woman of few words, but when she spoke she always had something very important to say. I recall her saying something along the lines of "give to others and you will receive tenfold in return." This adage has been at the heart of my focus in life and in my professional endeavors.

Let's face it, college, career, and life can be extremely competitive, but only if you insist on making it that way. It is important to be driven and have a life plan to guide you, but the beauty of life is to enjoy it with others and to experience the sense of accomplishment together.

My experiences as captain of a sports team, president of a fraternity, and a senior resident made me realize that a team of diverse individuals all moving toward the same goal was much better than a disparate group of folks striving for individual accomplishments. I determined that my professional focus would be best suited to lead a pharmacy team. To be a great pharmacist, it is essential to embrace leadership as a professional responsibility because you must lead on your patients' behalf; lead when working with nurses, physicians, and other health professionals to manage drug therapy; and lead your personal, professional journey.

So, can you imagine being 24 years old and your first job after completing a residency is assistant director of pharmacy in a children's hospital in Washington, DC, with staff representing almost every nationality reporting to you? Well, this long-haired, lily-white, young, residency-trained, hot shot was disdained by most of this extremely diverse staff. I was overwhelmed, constantly challenged, and quickly becoming worn down. Had I made a huge mistake? Could I handle the pressure? Did I believe in myself that I could be successful? Ultimately, after several nerve-racking months, I resorted to focusing on my core values of giving my best and believing that it would pay dividends—and indeed it did! I focused on serving patients with the utmost quality, respecting each individual's important contribution to the pharmacy team, and being totally honest and demonstrating integrity in all that I did. Guess what? It paid off ten times over. I became the Director of

Pharmacy, stayed in the organization 17 years, and was a preceptor to 45 residents. My reward was having patients' parents tell me how much they appreciated having their pharmacist oversee their child's chemotherapy regime, having doctors ask me when they could get a pharmacist on their care team, and most importantly, pharmacy residents and staff members giving 110 percent every day to do the right thing for our patients. Think about what you are willing to give as you begin your career and it will set the stage for reaping rewards later.

I cannot gloss over the vital impact of relationship development among pharmacy professionals and the need for mentorship. I was fortunate to have a pharmacy residency preceptor and a pharmacy director who hired me out of the residency invest in me at a critical time in my professional development. They helped launch my career, and I am indebted to them forever for my success. I took a cue from my mentors in becoming a preceptor, and undoubtedly, it has been the most fulfilling professional experience giving me immense pride and joy. My residents are my lifelong friends, and I live vicariously through their accomplishments. I suggest that you seek out a mentor(s) and recognize that you have the same responsibility to give back to other young professionals throughout your career.

Thus far I have talked mostly about work. But pharmacy is a profession and not just the place of employment where you just show up and serve patients. To be an effective professional, you must continually invest in your professional development. Professional organizations, such as state and national pharmacy associations, are fantastic stages for young practitioners to hone their leadership and practice skills. Early in my career, I was newly married, expecting our first child, and just appointed the director of pharmacy, when I suddenly became president-elect of the state hospital pharmacy organization. To make the situation more challenging, the association's president took a job in another state, and I was thrust into serving as president for two years. I was scared on the inside but had to demonstrate confidence and poise outwardly. By showing that I cared, working hard, and asking for help, I was amazed at the response and support I received. I made lifelong friendships and honed my organizational skills from that state association leadership experience. So, I suggest that you step out and step up and become a professional association participant and leader on a local and national level.

In case you think that my life ran smoothly, let me tell you that I had some dark professional moments and you likely will, too. At the time, these professional crises seemed to be earth-shattering. So, what are my dark moments? I was caught in a consultant's downsizing at the peak of my career. I lost my job and a 17-year career in one fell swoop. I was pushed out in the middle of the day, and I went home with my professional life turned upside down. I walked into my house; my daughter had never seen me home on a week day in the middle of the day and she was crushed to think that daddy was fired. I ultimately fared better than the other staff who lost their jobs because of my attitude and professional confidence. Following that devastating day, I had job offers and consulting opportunities due to the investment I made in my career. You should never lose faith in your professional abilities, take a deep breath, and think about how you will handle adversity. Remember to act with poise and confidence and rely on your professional network for support. Ultimately, how we handle adversity speaks to who we are and how we feel about our professional abilities.

I wish to relate one more disappointing professional encounter and describe how it turned out to be a fantastic opportunity. One of my lifelong professional goals was to be on the board of directors of ASHP—my national, professional organization. I had the opportunity to vie for an ASHP board position but lost the election. I was crushed, but it turned out to be a blessing in disguise. As an ASHP board member, I would have had the opportunity to give back to my profession by serving for a three-year period. In my mind it was the ultimate opportunity shy of being president of ASHP. But, it is difficult to become ASHP president if you can't get elected to the board. I thought that I was a washed-up volunteer association leader. Little did I know that a few key association leaders envisioned a different leadership opportunity for me. Five years later, I was invited to interview for ASHP Foundation's Chief Executive Officer position, and I am fortunate to serve our profession in that capacity. My full-time position is dedicated to advancing the role of the health-system pharmacist. What a gift these past 15 years have been. I am working every day to give back to those who will follow you and me in our profession!

In closing, keep in mind that whatever you invest in this profession of pharmacy, it will likely return to you in tenfold benefits.

*Steve*

# Ernest R. Anderson, Jr.

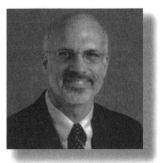

## *Stay True to Your Values*

You will never meet a more values-centered person than Ernie. He has an incredibly strong foundation in his faith, has built a very successful career as a servant leader, and is proud of his success in building supportive cultures allowing individuals to thrive. His faith and values have certainly guided him through challenging times when there were conflicts with his values in his work environment. Such experiences served to strengthen his commitment to his values and through his letter you will benefit from his experiences.

Ernie is the founder of Ernest R. Anderson, Jr. Consulting, Inc., and consults in all aspects of pharmacy practice with health-system pharmacies. He is formerly System Vice President of Pharmacy at Steward Health Care and has held various leadership positions in hospitals and health systems during his career. He is also Associate Clinical Professor of Pharmacy at Northeastern University College of Pharmacy and Allied Health Professions, and Adjunct Associate Professor of Pharmacy at Massachusetts College of Pharmacy and Health Sciences. He is also active in various professional organizations and is an author and national speaker on numerous leadership and pharmacy practice topics. He received his bachelor of science and master of science degrees from Northeastern University College of Pharmacy and Allied Health Professions.

Ernie shares that there will likely be times in your career that your values are challenged and encourages you to *carefully consider the values that are important to you and your life and stay true to them.*

Dear Young Pharmacist,

Y ou are uniquely gifted and when you utilize those gifts in your chosen career, working will be a privilege and a pleasure, not drudgery. Think carefully about the various aspects of your life and get a vision for each. Setting goals that align with your values is extremely important and will help you to have balance within all these aspects in concert with one another. Through balancing all areas of your life, you will increase your professional and personal satisfaction; however, you will, no doubt, experience challenging times in your career. Author Andy Andrews has stated: "We are either in a crisis, coming out of a crisis or going into a crisis." This is part of life. Let me share some of my challenging times, my lessons learned, and how I was guided by staying true to my values.

One difficulty was that it is impossible for me to compartmentalize who I am. In my first job I moved up the ranks into a pharmacy management position. I did well in this job for many years until conflicts arose with my boss over differences in our values. As a Christian, every aspect of my life is Christ centered. I was told to leave my "religion to Sundays." In our department, I was the go-to person that everyone consulted, and my council is derived from the Bible and other Christian mentors with a similar focus. I remember the head of our drug information center kidding with me that I always had a line at my door. My values were to care for people and help them be successful in their professional and personal lives. Although people valued my wisdom, which was largely based on Biblical principles, my boss did not. We had many discussions where I tried to explain that being precedes doing and I do what I do because I am what I am. I am a Christian. The bottom line, my values of sharing the love of Christ were not shared, and I was fired after 17 years at the hospital. I was devastated. I remember packing my office into boxes with tears in my eyes, while the locksmith was changing the lock on my door. The employees that I was leaving were my friends whom I cared for deeply. No one quite understood what went on. Some thought I left on my own accord, and they "respected my decision." When I arrived home,

I remember hugging my wife and daughter, crying and asking, What am I going to do now? Fortunately, I had two immediate advantages going for me. First, a good friend who was an outplacement counselor and, second, my faith community was incredibly supportive. With the help of my outplacement friend, I negotiated a severance package and an outplacement service and started looking for a job. My local network of professional friends was very supportive and helped me with references, job leads, and moral support. Within three months, I accepted a new job as pharmacy director. The lessons learned are the power of networking: when you help others, they are very willing to help you. And secondly, what I thought was hugely negative turned into a positive in that I moved to a new, higher level position.

In this new role as pharmacy director, our department established many innovative pharmacy programs. I continued to present lectures and posters, and became more involved in our local and national pharmacy societies. My extensive knowledge regarding financial management and reimbursement led to many speaking opportunities across the country. I regarded this as a method to serve my profession. Through this service attitude my leadership grew. I continue to find servant leadership to be the best type of leadership. Jesus demonstrated and spoke about being a servant to all.

Unfortunately, the misalignment of values occurred twice more in my career. Although our pharmacy department became nationally recognized, my new boss could not understand why I wanted to pursue an elected office to serve the American Society of Health-System Pharmacists (ASHP). There was no recognition for the importance of networking with colleagues in pharmacy to advance the profession. Once again, I experienced a situation where my values did not align with those of my boss. However, this time I decided to leave to be true to my values. Pursuing national office was a professional goal that would not be supported at my current job. After praying and agonizing, I left to pursue a vice-president of pharmacy position in a multi-hospital system. I learned, as you will also, to own my values and my career.

My new boss was supportive of my national recognition. We shared values of the importance of national service and networking. All was fine until our system was bought by a capital investment company and became a for-profit organization. Eventually, my position was eliminated in a cost reduction initiative. I viewed this event very differently than I had the first time I was let go. The circumstances were very different, but the outcome the same. This time I was in charge of my career, and I saw it as a divine opportunity to pursue something new. Within a few months, I developed my own consulting company, and I am very much enjoying my work.

As I look back over my career, it is obvious how important it is for me to work in an environment where my values align with those around me. As you consider employment opportunities, I advise you to

- Assess how your values will align with a person or organization as you consider a job.

- Construct a personal mission statement that enumerates your values. This will become your guidepost as you seek employment throughout your career.

- Determine if your values line up with the prospective new employer during the interview process by questioning this potential employer.

- Be specific about the pharmacy values and the personal values of the pharmacy leader. This goes beyond the values of the organization.

My faith in a loving God pervades everything that I do. As I study leadership books and articles, I find the principles related there are not new. In fact they are quite old. The Bible is an historical living word that is the basis for every leadership principle that I read and study.

An adage that I often teach is "Being precedes doing. We do what we do because we are what we are." This is all about character.

The characteristics that I believe have been most useful are:

- exercising a strong work ethic,

- having a mentor and be a mentor,

- sharing your knowledge, and

- living your faith as a servant leader,

This will help to build your network. Volunteer in societies and organizations and practice leadership principles to enhance your relationships and serve others. As you grow professionally and perhaps move into leadership positions, strive to make others successful. Then you will be successful, too.

Sincerely,
*Ernie Anderson*

# Roberta M. Barber

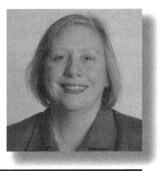

## *Just How Do You Know When to Make a Job Move?*

When you meet Roberta, you will find an energetic dynamo who encountered and solved the challenges of balancing and integrating a successful leadership career with raising two children as a single parent. While there is not just one way to handle these challenges, she describes the trade-offs, which are so important to take into account—including the things to consider when you feel your job is not working out. Roberta identifies what an appropriate job fit really means.

Roberta completed her bachelor of science and doctor of pharmacy degrees at Union University Albany College of Pharmacy and her master's of public health at Columbia University's Joseph Mailman School of Public Health. Roberta is currently Assistant Vice President of Pharmacy Services, Virtua Health System in New Jersey.

In her letter, she states, *your career may take a winding career path; taking the risk and finding the courage to move from one job to another, but experiencing great joy, satisfaction, and reward in the journey.*

Dear Young Pharmacist,

Y ou should be very proud of your career choice to practice pharmacy. On occasion, I have been asked why I selected pharmacy. In high school, I had a love for both chemistry and music. Eventually, I made my decision by process of elimination, with some family support. My mother was very influential in my decision;

not having had a career herself, she wanted her daughters to pursue a profession. I felt drawn to health care, and pharmacy seemed to rise to the top, and it is a decision that I have not regretted. I tell you this because it is just the beginning of all the decisions and choices you will make as you progress through your career, and how you go about making these choices is just as important as the result.

Pharmacy is a profession which offers a wide variety of practice venues. Whether it is industry, academia, clinical research, nuclear pharmacy, compounding pharmacy, retail or hospital pharmacy, there is something for every personality type and for every stage of your career. Many choose one type of practice and remain in that area for their entire career and that is fine. However, there are far too many opportunities in pharmacy to be dissatisfied or unhappy for too long in any job. So if you feel this way, it is time to start exploring your options.

I can honestly say that after 32 years of pharmacy practice, I still love my profession. Although times have changed during my years as a pharmacist, there still are some commonalities and consistencies. I have made several moves in my career: each time advancing my practice and knowledge base, each time with gratifying results.

So, you may ask, just how do I know when to make a move in my job or career? Sometimes it can be a difficult decision, but I will attempt to outline some guiding principles I use in my decision making. Some reasons you may consider a job change:

- More challenge or sense of accomplishment
- Positioning for promotion and/or advancement
- Better job "fit"

So how do you know it is time to consider something new or different?

- When you feel you have accomplished all you can in your current position, and there is nothing else that you can contribute to the organization, department, or your job.
- If you feel you need a more stimulating and challenging environment, and you need to feel more satisfaction at the end of the day.
- When you feel you have no room for advancement, and that is something you desire, and you have researched all available opportunities.

- When after giving it a good try, you determine it is a "no-win" situation or the environment is not supporting your goals and/or values.

- When you feel that your talents could be better utilized in another arena, and there is just no way to express them in your current situation.

At times it is necessary to consider a job change for the purpose of positioning. If you have an interest or goal to become a leader or move up the leadership ladder, you may need to change jobs or roles within your current organization or find a new position elsewhere. This can sometimes get tricky. At times it is more art than science, but many corporate executives do it and it is a well-known tactic to build a resume for career growth. For example, I left a perfectly solid, secure, good-paying job as a director to take a job in a larger hospital, for the same money, farther away from my home. The new hospital was mostly unknown to me, but I saw the move as an opportunity to position myself for the next stage of my career. It was a huge growth period for me, but it was not without *sacrifice*. The change meant more time away from my home and children with the longer commute and more focus on my job. So, what does sacrifice mean to you? This is something you will have to determine for yourself.

Last, but not least, there is the matter of "fit" for a job. Fit, to me, means that the individual's personality and other preferences align well with the job requirements and type of work expected. It is important to explore your options and think about the different environments in which you feel comfortable. You can get a feel for the various work environments while you are on your rotations; keeping in mind, of course, that it is much different being a student on rotation than experiencing the same environment as a real-world pharmacist. Nonetheless, the rotations can help you in making your career choice. Another way to establish fit is to explore various settings by working as a student/technician in a hospital, retail, or industrial setting.

You need to ask yourself how important a better lifestyle, or work/ life balance and fit is for you. I can honestly say I did not examine the concept of fit at the time I took that position at the larger hospital, but I soon realized that the job was very demanding. Fortunately, I loved it, so I needed to come to terms with how to deal with the demand it was placing on my life. It took a lot of time management (juggling), commitment, and prioritization. I made a trade-off—a full time job to support my family and the directorship that would provide me with professional satisfaction and the opportunity to learn and grow at the expense of more limited family time.

Sometimes fit means considering if a job may demand a characteristic or an attribute that you have not yet developed, or even something that you have no interest in. When I was learning the ropes in management, I found myself in positions that were too demanding for me at that point in my life or professional development. As much as I sacrificed, it never seemed to be enough to do the job the way it needed to be done. Conversely, I have also had jobs where the culture was not ready for the change that I was well prepared to lead. In both cases, the "fit" was not right.

At some point, hopefully early in your career, there will be an "Aha" moment—a moment or time when it all comes together and you know the right pharmacy path to take. I generally like to think through decisions as serious as a job change; however, I can honestly say that some decisions are so obvious that the faster you move on, the better off you will be!

You will find your niche. It may be your current job offers all you need to develop and grow. Or you may be like me, on a winding career path; taking risks and finding the courage to move from one job to another, and experiencing great joy, satisfaction, and reward in the journey. Either way, best of luck and good fortune to you as you find your path and fit!

*Roberta M. Barber*

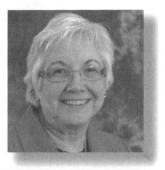

# Marialice S. Bennett

## *It Takes a Team to Create Change*

Marialice ventured into clinical pharmacy at its inception in the 1970s, learning as she went because clinical education and clinical residencies were just beginning. She was indeed a pioneer and risk taker. Her career has focused on instituting new clinical practices and training residents and pharmacy students. She has continued to be innovative in creating, implementing, and conducting Community and Ambulatory Pharmacy Residency programs as well as cofounding, with a physician, an employee interprofessional wellness health clinic (University Health Connection). Marialice is one of only a few women who have served as president of American Pharmacists Association (APhA).

She completed her bachelor of science in pharmacy at The Ohio State University College of Pharmacy. Marialice is currently Professor Emeritus, College of Pharmacy, The Ohio State University, and Director of the Community and Ambulatory Care Residency Program.

In her letter she states that there were times it was necessary to ask forgiveness rather than permission in creating a new practice and that *it would not have happened if we had followed all the politically correct channels.*

Dear Young Pharmacist,

Some would say I am a pioneer. I would say I am a risk taker. I don't believe I have ever had an original idea. But I have always been able to "catch" an idea and then make something innovative or creative happen. Motivational speaker Joel Barker says, "Vision without action is just a dream. Action without vision just passes the time. Vision with action can change the world." One must take risks to do all three. One must take risks to become an agent of change.

I had the amazing opportunity to become one of the first clinical pharmacists in the country in the early 1970s. I completed my internship at The Ohio State University Medical Center during a time when intravenous admixture programs, unit dose dispensing, and pharmacy liaisons to the nursing units were introduced as pilot projects. When I returned to the medical center as a pharmacist, I opened the ninth and tenth floors to unit dose dispensing and technician administration of medications, and I began creating clinical pharmacists' roles on the nursing unit and on medical teams. It was a magical journey with magical people. Our administrative staff made us believe we could be agents of change even though we had not been trained for the new roles we were creating. Even though we were taking high-stake risks, we believed in ourselves, in each other, and in the new evolving roles for pharmacists.

There were times in the early years of clinical pharmacy when doing the right thing for the patient was very risky. As I reflect back, I had guiding principles that directed my risk-taking activities. I had managed to gain enough trust to begin to round with the medical teams on both the renal service and the renal transplant service. I remember holding an inappropriately high dose of gentamicin on a patient with renal failure because I could not find any one who was willing to change the order of the attending physician on the renal transplant service. The fellow from a renal service told me, "You know what you need to do." So I chose to hold the evening dose. The next morning, the attending physician was irate and refused to allow me to round any more on his service. That was OK—I did what I knew I needed to do. Three months later I was personally paged by that same attending physician to dose one of his patients in renal failure on methicillin, and I was welcomed back to the team. I have always felt that the moment when I did what I knew I needed to do for that patient was the moment I became a clinical pharmacist.

Many opportunities grew from the "back door" approach of creating trust and building relationships with other health care providers. Finding physician champions was key to my success in creating change. Supporting medical students and interns during their training led to strong partnerships when those same practitioners became residents and attending physicians. Making solid recommendations, researching difficult questions, and assisting the team whenever possible led to opportunities to become part of the team, start new programs, and create teaching rotations for residents and students.

Ultimately, using a "front door" approach of collaboration and innovation enabled us to open University Health Connection as an interprofessional practice. I met a physician in the 1990s who believed strongly in the collaboration and innovation. She was practicing as a physician in an urgent care clinic for faculty and staff down the hall from the Outpatient Pharmacy and was also involved in creating a wellness program for the university. I was practicing out of the Outpatient Pharmacy as a clinical faculty member creating pharmacy-provided patient care services and a new residency program in community care. As our relationship grew, the first community residents and I began to practice in her clinic and in the wellness program. Together, we saw the need for a worksite clinic for faculty and staff based on a wellness model. In 1999, we opened University Health Connection in the college of pharmacy with five people —a physician, a pharmacist, a nurse, a pharmacy technician, and an office associate. Almost 15 years later, the clinic now has over 18 employees, provides primary care, urgent care, bridge care, and wellness services for employees and has integrated multiple health care providers onto the interprofessional team. It also serves as a training site for students of multiple disciplines and both post-graduate year one and two (PGY1 and PGY2) residency programs. The medical director can still frequently be heard saying, "I love my pharmacists!" She is one of the greatest advocates for pharmacist-provided patient care services and the pharmacist role on the patient care team within and outside of our practice.

It became obvious that partnering with people with complementary skill sets gave sustainability to the ideas that I would "catch." I learned quickly that I am good at creating and implementing, but I am a very poor maintainer. I am not good at getting down in the weeds and become bored easily without the challenges of creating. Tools such as *Strengths Finder* and *Myers-Briggs Type Indicator* help identify your own strengths and give you great clues to identify the skill set you need for strong potential partners. It takes a team to create change —a well-thought-out team of players with complementary skill sets to make a dream come true. The medical director of University Health Connection and I had great vision and perseverance to create it, but it took the skill sets of our amazing staff to make it run like a fine-tuned machine and to function well within the university.

Making sure you are doing the right thing, having the right partners, and creating the vision and action plan are key to winning over support and ultimately gaining permission. Pushing the envelope to create change requires risk taking and does not always follow the traditional pathway of doing things. Of course, there were times when it seemed necessary to ask forgiveness rather than permission. Change is difficult for almost everyone. Each time I have been involved in creating a new practice, it would not have happened if we had followed all of the politically correct channels.

If I have a regret, it would be that I did not become more involved in advocacy earlier in my career. I feel like I have always been an advocate for the patient and the profession in my everyday work life. But I left the work of promoting our profession to the government and outside stakeholders to our state and national leadership. I began to recognize during our fight to have the privilege to administer immunizations how important advocacy is to how we practice every day. To move medication therapy management, the Affordable Care Act, and pharmacists as providers forward, it is so important for all stakeholders including patients, health care providers, payers, employers, legislators, and other organizations outside of pharmacy, to hear our message and to hear the stories of the patients we have impacted. To make an impact at this level requires active participation in state and national pharmacy organizations for all of us throughout our entire careers. We must be at the table with decision makers to keep our profession alive and to continue to impact the patients we serve.

So my message to you would be to get involved, stay involved, and "catch" an idea! Find some small or large way to become a change agent to secure the future of pharmacy and to provide better care for our patients. Lead from where you stand today and grow into a mentor and leader for the pharmacists of tomorrow. Together we can make a difference!

Sincerely,
*Marialice Bennett*

# Susan Teil Boyer

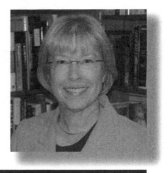

## *You Need the Big E: Enthusiasm*

Just ask Susan and she will tell you that knowing what you want to accomplish coupled with an enthusiastic drive to make it happen will get you a long way down the path of success. Susan's natural enthusiasm in her work and throughout her life has certainly been a key to her success.

Her pharmacy practice roots are in hospitals where she advanced the practice of pharmacy in hospitals of various sizes. She has served in several pharmacy and hospital administration leadership roles including Vice President and Director, Pharmacy Services, MultiCare Health System, Tacoma and Puyallup, Washington. She has also provided leadership on regulatory matters as Executive Director of the Washington State Board of Pharmacy. Throughout her career she has positively impacted the pharmacy profession in numerous roles and has always been an inspiration in developing residency programs and mentorship of residents. Thus, it is no surprise that she continues this passion for residency training and mentorship through her current role as Lead Surveyor for the ASHP Residency Accreditation Services Division. Susan also enjoys giving back to the pharmacy profession through her leadership in state and national pharmacy organizations including serving on the American Society of Health-System Pharmacists (ASHP) Board of Directors.

She received her bachelor of science degree from the University of Washington and her master of science degree from The Ohio State University where she also completed her residency in Pharmacy Practice and Administration. Susan tells us: *if you are going to advance your career or your cause you need to have enthusiasm.*

Dear Young Pharmacist,

In your training you learn all about drugs, but your profession is really about people, especially your patients. The most important thing for you is to relate to other people. Relating to others is about interacting effectively with a diverse range of people, the ability to listen actively, recognize different points of view, negotiate, and share ideas. Everything you wish for in your professional life will likely come from or through another person.

In my first year of a two-year pharmacy residency program at The Ohio State University (OSU) Medical Center, my preceptor, Dr. Clif Latiolais, said "Susan you have the big *E*, enthusiasm!" The words stuck with me, and my interest in others and interest in the profession carried me through several jobs and through increasing levels of professional involvement. Five years after graduating, I had the opportunity to take a director job in the Pacific North West at a multi-hospital community health system. I believe the big *E* came through for me as we enthusiastically worked to reshape our pharmacy practice model by convincing my boss and nursing leaders to decentralize the pharmacists to clinically practice on the patient care units. What a positive experience for the staff and for patient care! Enthusiasm ensures that you come across as someone who wants to do what it takes to get the job done.

Of course, some of our pharmacists were very excited to work on the patient care units and others, not so much. Change can be difficult, but enthusiasm helped me go above and beyond to stay committed to our vision. Ultimately, with time, the staff all supported our vision for care and services.

An important example I want to share with you was the opportunity I had to hire a new pharmacist. I looked for those intangibles where it boils down to experience versus enthusiasm; to me, enthusiasm wins every day of the week. Sure, training and experience are important, but we were sending the pharmacists to practice on the nursing units so it was important that the new pharmacist had energy, enthusiasm, optimism, and resilience.

Enthusiasm also helped me get along with other managers—even difficult ones—and respond to their needs with optimism, maturity, and a willingness to improve. Another example was my introduction to a new nurse manager in the intensive care unit (ICU). I explained that we were placing a clinical pharmacist in ICU, but since she had no experience with this model, she pushed back with little understanding of the pharmacist's role. I met with her several times, and I believe my passionate interest in helping the nursing staff, patients, and physicians convinced her to support our plan. Eventually, the nurse manager became our biggest ally for decentralized services!

Find your big *E*—your enthusiasm—and share it with others. Your interest in others will come through because your goal is not to be right but to do the right thing by others. Your interest and enthusiasm will open doors for you that you might not expect.

Accept that you continue to grow, develop, and change. You cannot really predict who you will be or where your path will take you several years from now. I do know you will be a different person. The Ohio State University residency program put me into a network of graduates of the program, pharmacy leaders, and mentors. I had no idea when I started the program I would travel the path I did. Director and assistant director jobs were not available where I lived. So instead of finding my first post-residency job in Seattle, I interviewed for a job in Denver for a leadership role. I met an OSU graduate and director of pharmacy who became a mentor and was willing to hire me. They were looking for someone who demonstrated enthusiasm, cooperation, and a willingness to work hard. From this position I began building my experience and future professional career. You really do not know what lies ahead in five or 10 years. Make the effort to get to know your colleagues in and out of your hospital/health system. They may help you down your path. Be open and ready to take advantage of opportunities.

By networking and building relationships, you invite broader possibilities as your career develops. Pharmacy and certainly health-system pharmacy is a small profession—someone will know someone else who knows you and your work. Share your support and advice; these connections will keep you going during frustrating times. In fact, networking can increase your job options and opportunities so that you find yourself down a new pharmacy path. I joined the Washington state board of pharmacy as a hospital/health-system member in 2000. The state board membership allowed me to participate more broadly in the profession—to make a difference. After eight years as a member on the state board, I was recruited to the executive director position, never dreaming this would be a career option for me. Again, be open to the possibilities! There are many paths in pharmacy. By getting involved in the profession, you will find so many benefits.

Develop your big *E*, follow your heart, relate to others, network, and get involved in the profession!

Best wishes to you.

Sincerely,
*Susan Teil Boyer*

# Richard D. Caldwell

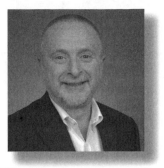

## *Venture Out of Your Comfort Zone*

Fun and adventuresome are two words that will come to mind when you meet Richard. As you will read, he enjoys new opportunities and is often in search of new knowledge and experiences to satisfy his sense of adventure. International travel is one source of adventure for Richard. In his current role, he travels the globe experiencing and learning new cultures, has first-hand observations of health care and pharmacy practice in foreign lands, shares his pharmacy knowledge and experience, and, of course, enjoys the international food.

Richard is now Senior Manager for International Markets for Omnicell directing global marketing efforts and providing consultations. He specializes in patient safety, workflow optimization, and pharmacy and nurse efficiency associated with medication automation. Prior to joining Omnicell, he was Associate Director and subsequent Director of Pharmacy Services at Stanford Hospital & Clinics in Palo Alto, California, and has held leadership and clinical positions in community and university hospitals. He also holds faculty appointments at several Colleges of Pharmacy, including University of California at San Francisco, University of Pacific, Albany College of Pharmacy, and Touro University.

Richard's education and training journey began in his home state of North Carolina with a bachelor of science degree from the University of North Carolina at Chapel Hill; residency at Lutheran General Hospital in Park Ridge, Illinois; and a master of science degree and residency at the University of Kansas. Richard tells us, *don't be afraid to venture out of your comfort zone.*

Dear Young Pharmacist,

Your goals of an education and stable career probably seem reachable to you at this point in your life, but do your dreams seem more impossible? I encourage you to dream and allow yourself to imagine what might seem impossible to you now. Then venture outside your comfort zone and follow your dreams. With clarity of goals and dreams you will find alignment and discover opportunities that are not obvious to you today. Let me share my story.

I grew up in rural North Carolina in a town of 300 or so. To this day it remains a small town, although surrounded by increasing growth. Growing up, my exposure to the world was as limited as the handful of channels on our old Magnavox black and white console television set. I remember at an early age thinking that there must be more to the world than what I knew, and so I began to dream of the possibilities.

I knew I was different than other kids where I grew up. I always wanted more than was available to me. I just knew there was more, and I was determined to look for it. Most people where I lived never moved away. They stayed, raised families, and worked locally. This was a very good thing, for them, but not me. I wanted to travel and experience the world. The idea of living in different places was intriguing and exciting. Once I came to terms with my goals of a stable career and a future of exploration and learning about the world, I set out to do just that. Pharmacy has allowed me to do exactly what I set out to do. Although I didn't initially set out to simultaneously achieve both my career path and my dreams of seeing the world, I subconsciously did just that through my choices and the options presented to me. My goals and my dreams were aligned. My journey was and is about having a solid career that allows you to follow your dreams.

I entered the university and applied to pharmacy school after my first year. I was accepted and started the 4-year path to complete my bachelor of science degree. During my senior experiential year, I was able to complete a rotation in a rural health clinic about one hour from the university and carpooled with the preceptor. During these weekly rides, he questioned me on my post-graduate plans, introducing me to the idea of completing a residency. These conversations with the preceptor coupled with my summer internship as a medication assistant (medication nurse) at a university hospital convinced me that hospital pharmacy would be my career path. It seemed to coincide well with my aspirations and life goals. I purposely applied to residency programs that were out-of-state allowing me to move to a different part of the country and see pharmacy practice in a different view and begin my journey.

I moved to Chicago and started a 1-year residency program. Coming from a town of 300 people to Chicago, you can imagine how my whole being awakened to the possibilities that lay ahead. After my few but rewarding years in Chicago and with the director of pharmacy's encouragement, I decided to apply to joint master of science/residency programs, moving me yet again. This time to Kansas City followed by a position as Assistant Director of Pharmacy in a South Carolina hospital. From my beginnings in the rural south to the big Midwest city, to the plains, and then back in the South, I had come full circle but I was still not satisfied. Yet another opportunity came as a director of pharmacy position in South Florida, which exposed me to a diverse community that began to look more like the world I imagined. There were Hispanics, Jews, African Americans, and Europeans. A plethora of languages and cultures, not unlike what I got a taste of in Chicago, except this experience had palm trees and beaches, miles of white sand, the bluest of skies, and never-ending summers. I was OK with my life at this point. I had a stable job and was helping and meeting all kinds of different people. My South Florida experience was beginning to have an influence on me culturally, politically, and personally. Yet I thirsted for more.

From South Florida, I moved to Northern California where the final installment of my journey as a hospital pharmacist has come to fruition. In California, I had the opportunity to get involved in pharmacy automation. Clearly, my career as a pharmacist was evolving into something quite different from what I had originally envisioned, but evolving nicely into the life that I always imagined. The knowledge base I had gained to this point coupled with my increasing interests in other aspects of the field led to a position with an automation company. After 25 years of hospital practice, I made the leap. This new adventure allowed me to use my pharmacy knowledge and required me to travel and assist in implementation optimization of automation throughout the United States. I had the best of both worlds—working as a pharmacist and the opportunity to experience more of my world. My goals and dreams were continuing to align.

The ability to work with different pharmacists, understand their needs for patient care, and represent those needs to my company has been immensely rewarding. After five years, I was given the opportunity to move to the international division. It was a bit overwhelming at first as I understood U.S. pharmacy, but now I was venturing outside to a world that I did not really know; however, the excitement of learning and the desire to experience more was now at my fingertips. Again, I was ready. The last four years of my career have been amazing. I have been fortunate to travel and work beside pharmacists from all five continents, understand our similarities and differences, and represent their needs in our changing world. From Chile to China, Saudi Arabia to Singapore and Qatar to Spain, the journey has been all that I hoped for and more. Walking along the Great Wall of China, driving through Patagonia—these are the experiences I always dreamed of. It is not without much personal sacrifice, however. It has meant 14-day trips away from my family, working in environments completely foreign to me, communicating through interpreters, learning to eat strange foods, and adhering to different and wonderful customs like flying alongside hundreds of Muslims traveling to Mecca.

The professional satisfaction of feeling like a true citizen of this amazing world we live in has been a dream come true for me. I have learned first-hand that pharmacists are not all that different worldwide—we are much more alike than not. Our goal of safe patient care is consistent no matter where I have traveled.

Here is what I have learned and what I hope you will learn:

- Don't be afraid to venture out of your comfort zone.

- Allow yourself to evolve as a pharmacist, as a person.

- Come to terms with your goals and your dreams and do not hesitate to take on new roles and responsibilities that align with your personal and professional interest. Explore and design your own path.

- Learn from all that surrounds you, your mentors, and those you meet along your journey.
- Be the best you can be and live your dreams.

Respectfully yours,
*Richard Caldwell*

# Susan A. Cantrell

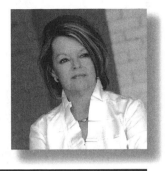

## *We Can Have It All, We Just Can't Always Do It All*

You can easily spot Susan across the room at a meeting as she is always one of the best-dressed! Her competence is more than appearance, however. She has successfully integrated marriage, raising two children, and her career. While at the American Society of Health-System Pharmacists (ASHP), she and her team developed, and successfully grew ASHP Advantage, which specializes in conducting cutting-edge continuing educational programs. Susan has always been an innovator, adopting new technology such as podcasts, webinars, and electronic audience feedback, into educational programs to improve the profession.

Exploring new leadership vistas outside of pharmacy, Susan is currently the Senior Vice President and Managing Director of DIA Americas with the Drug Information Association (DIA), a global, nonprofit association that provides knowledge resources across the full spectrum of medical product development and fosters innovation to improve health and well-being worldwide.

Susan received her bachelor of science in pharmacy from the University of Mississippi and completed a residency at the University of Mississippi Medical Center. Susan's letter offers the following advice: *When faced with difficult decisions that place your personal or family interests at odds with your career, the best you can do is make sure to give equal consideration to career and personal factors when making career choices and deal with the guilt about missing the dance recital, soccer game, or the important budget meeting.*

Dear Young Pharmacist,

You have chosen your career wisely! In addition to the personal and professional fulfillment you will receive from helping patients throughout your career, the practice of pharmacy offers you so many career opportunities. At some point in your career, you will likely be faced with a difficult decision that places your personal or family interests at odds with those of your career. These decisions are intensely personal, but I will share some insights from my own career that I hope will help you.

I was drawn to pharmacy by my first "real" job, a clerk in a local community pharmacy during high school. I loved the community pharmacy environment and envisioned myself graduating from pharmacy school and working part-time in a community pharmacy while raising a family. My career aspirations shifted during my last year of pharmacy school when I did an experiential rotation in a hospital pharmacy department. Hospital practice intrigued and excited me and the director of pharmacy, an experienced and capable female leader, served as a strong role model. I was hooked.

As luck would have it, during that rotation I learned about a new hospital pharmacy residency program at University of Mississippi Medical Center, which could prepare me for my intended career in hospital pharmacy. I was very motivated to apply; however, I was a new mother with an infant son born the week classes began in my final year of pharmacy school. Just getting through that final year would be a significant challenge. The idea of committing to a year of residency with the stress of being the only resident and the first resident admitted to the program and working a 12-days-on, 2-days-off schedule was daunting. This was the first of many decisions I would have to make where my career and family interests were seemingly juxtaposed.

I do not remember exactly what factors tipped the scale, but I decided that residency training was the right path for me. Although it would be difficult, I had a support system of family and friends to get me through it. Even though I would be earning less than half of what most of my classmates were being offered, it seemed like a prudent investment in my career. Looking back so many years later, I can say without hesitation that it was the right decision for me, both professionally and personally. It was a tough year, and there were times when I was not sure if I could finish the year. There were also many times I felt I had to skimp on my parenting duties to fulfill my job's expectations. Unfortunately, that is true of anyone who has a career and a family. We can *have* it all, we just can't always *do* it all. The best we can do is make sure we give equal consideration to career and personal factors when making our career choices and deal with the guilt we will no doubt feel along the way about missing the dance recital, soccer game, or the important budget meeting.

My loving and supportive husband and partner has made my decisions about career and family easier. Like many couples, we have had challenging careers throughout our marriage that necessitated extended and frequent travel, long hours, and geographic relocations. Unlike many couples, we have a partnership where responsibilities and decision-making are shared and stereotypical roles are irrelevant. When our children were growing up, one of us would step in when the other could not. While I wish I could take the credit for establishing this paradigm, I have to confess that it all goes to my husband who set this ground rule   and this stellar example—so long ago.

Please do not think that this letter is intended to advise you about work-life balance; it surely is not. In fact, I avoid using that phrase at all. What comes to mind when I think of the word *balance* is the scale used in compounding medications, where you put a weight on one side of the scale and heap something on the other side so that the two sides weigh the same and balance is achieved. Well, maybe that works for pharmacy compounding, but I don't think it works for life situations. What happens if the scale is balanced but there is too much on both sides? Perhaps *work-life integration* is a better term, suggesting that one is able to combine work and personal life in a way that feels comfortable.

There have been times when I have fallen short on the work-life integration scale. Fortunately for me, my family does not remember those times when career trumped family considerations. But there are several examples I will always carry with me. Early in my tenure at ASHP, I was assigned to represent the organization at a meeting when my husband would also be traveling. Both of us traveling at the same time was not unusual, and we had an outstanding grandmotherly babysitter who could cover in these situations. The day before I departed, our younger son, a sixth-grader, lost a close friend to a rare chronic pulmonary disease. They had remained close during the friend's illness, and our son had visited him just days before his death. He was heartbroken. The funeral was to take place while I was away, so I had a decision to make. Our son's teacher offered to accompany him and a few other classmates to the funeral. After much deliberation, I decided to travel to the important meeting. Looking back, I know it was not the right decision and almost 20 years later, I still feel guilty. Our son vividly remembers the pain and sadness of the loss of his friend. However, when we spoke about it a few years ago, he did not remember feeling abandoned during this time of need. That our children still love us in spite of our shortcomings is both remarkable and fortuitous!

It is possible—and I certainly wish for you—that you will sail through your career, with each change being a positive one, on a smooth path to achieving your vision of personal and professional fulfillment. Unfortunately, that doesn't always happen and, along the way, you will likely have to make some tough decisions. Be prepared to make tough decisions about integrating your work and personal life. Be prepared for setbacks, but do not let them paralyze you when they occur. Try to overcome the guilt when you occasionally veer off the right path.

I wish you success, happiness, and prosperity,
*Susan Cantrell*

# Toby Clark

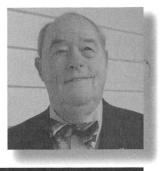

## *What Are You Going to Do for the Rest of Your Life?*

In addition to being a servant and skilled formal Big L leader, Toby continues to be committed to educating and training young people and as such is a consummate mentor as his letter outlines. He is an example of being extremely influential as a little "L" leader in professional organizations having worked to assist informatics practitioners to achieve their own American Society of Health-System Pharmacists (ASHP) Section. What is less obvious as you get to know him is he is an avid sailor who has sailed his boats up and down the East Coast for decades. Toby brings to his mentoring over 45 years of leadership and pharmacy teaching experience in both community and academic medical centers.

Toby received his bachelor of science in pharmacy degree from Ohio Northern University and his master of science degree from Wayne State University. He completed a residency at Bronson Methodist Hospital. He is currently an ASHP Residency Program Lead Surveyor and Practice Management Consultant.

In his letter he gives the following great advice: *One of the things that I learned is that an outward projection with a smile on one's face as well as a happy hello works well in all human relations.*

Dear Young Pharmacist,

Your graduation event was very well attended, and you were very privileged to hear an inspiring speaker. Although I have known you for the past three years, it was fascinating to speak with your parents after the graduation ceremony. They are as proud of all your accomplishments as am I. As one of your mentors, it has been my privilege to see you grow and expand your capabilities as you become a caregiver to patients. You asked me to summarize some of our discussions of the past years and project into the future a little.

Here is the question I pose for you. *What are you going to do for the rest of your life?* That question is coupled with another real thinker: *When will you retire?* The answers to those questions form the real basis of my personal thinking and reflections. Through our discussions, you have also learned to ask yourself, *What are my goals and how can I plan on reaching them?* As you know, only you can answer these questions. I have posed them in different ways to make you think about your answers as you complete your pharmacy education. Your life and your career are your responsibility. You cannot ask anyone else to live your life or pursue your career. We have talked about the value of post-graduate training until you did not wish to hear, read, or listen to me any more. But you are a smart person and you, by choosing to live a frugal life while in pharmacy school, kept your debt level low. That choice has now given you more options than many of your classmates who may drive newer cars, have taken vacations, wear more expensive clothes, but now have high debts to pay off. The wisdom of your no-credit-card debt philosophy will now pay dividends.

You have chosen to further develop your skills by completing a post-graduate year one residency. That decision will pay off greatly in your becoming a more competent pharmacist as you enter the work place. The added year of skill building and training will be very beneficial to you. We discussed at length the fact that you are giving up about $60,000 of salary to get this added training. But this year of training prepares you to have options that many of your peers will not have. You can decide to get another year of training in a post-graduate year two program and become an expert or you can go on to a career-objective position knowing that you have training that others lack. Because you are a goal-oriented person you may even seek graduate training in management or in some other clinical aspect.

You will be better prepared to serve because of your investment in yourself. You already know that being satisfied and confident in your career is more valuable than the dollars you missed when in training. You cannot place a monetary value or a return on investment on career satisfaction. There is no greater satisfaction than waking up each morning liking yourself for the way you live your life and the decisions you have made.

Your ability to reflect and deliberate the pros and cons of your decisions will be your foundation to build future feelings of confidence. You will continue to explore what you are good at and what you like to do. Reflection has taught you what your strengths really are and how to improve them. Remember, this is a never-ending process. No doubt, you will make some judgmental errors that will cause you to stop, rethink, and change your course of action. Mistakes will be made, but hopefully you will use those as learning experiences to help you find other opportunities for improvement.

Effectiveness in communication, relationship building, persistence, listening, and serving other people will enhance the mission and personal purpose you have set for yourself. How you treat other people is a very important value in your career. As you move from this period of intense education and training you will need to learn to work with other people. You are going to be working with people in the future that you would not socialize with whatsoever. No one says you need to have dinner or go to a movie with each and every person you work with. So keep in mind, and even force yourself if you must, to be polite and nice to everyone—all the time. Even sometimes in situations you abhor!

For you to optimize all of your experiences in pharmacy school and post-doctoral residency training and even graduate school, you need to constantly seek to apply your training to be effective with others. I strongly suggest that you never, ever make a decision that you do not like a patient. The choice of who you like and don't like and who you serve is not part of the professional's prerogative. Serve all patients who come your way. The same concept applies to everyone you work with day in and day out. It took me a while to learn this when I was a young hospital pharmacist. But when I did, and truly put it into play, it made my work time much simpler. Serve all and try extra hard to work with all.

A positive outward and inner attitude will play an important role in your everyday interactions with others. Through our discussions I have learned that even on the darkest of days you are an optimist at heart. You have learned to project the attitude that the glass is always more than half full. Through the years what has benefitted me a great deal has been the way of thinking that I can affect many people if I have a positive attitude and project that to them. In my experience it is the little things that I have learned that have made a big difference in my actions and reactions from others. One of the things I have also learned is that outward projection with a smile on one's face as well as a happy greeting works wonders in all human relations. By being an upbeat and "can do" person you can accomplish more than you thought possible. Believe in yourself and believe the best can be reached by a positive attitude.

Your ability to lead, serve, and give hope to others are values to embrace as you embark on your career. Although you had only a smattering of leadership training in pharmacy school, from our discussions I know you value what you have learned. Constantly strive to improve your leadership capabilities. You have the capacity and responsibility to lead yourself and others as you serve patients.

You are developing the attitude of service to others as part of your personal and professional values. This is already serving you well in your approach to others as evidenced by your leadership positions in your college professional organizations. Your accomplishment in this regard is outstanding. Your attitude of service to others was also evident in your recent residency interviews. Congratulations on obtaining your choice of residency in the recent match process. Others are already valuing your contributions because of your attitude and service philosophy.

Well, my friend, I trust this brief letter helps you to understand some of the discussions we have had these past few years. It has been my pleasure to mentor you. Now it is your turn to pass it forward.

I look forward to visiting with you at our next professional association meeting.

Cheers to your accomplishments,
*Toby Clark*

# Daniel J. Cobaugh

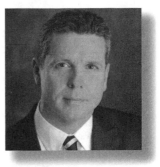

## *Love Being Exactly Who You Are*

You will likely leave your first encounter with Dan impressed by the charismatic and sincere person he is. You will find him very engaging and obviously someone who is appropriately confident and comfortable in his own skin. Arriving at his current state of self-confidence and comfort with himself was, however, a long and sometimes challenging journey. In the following letter, Dan explains that his strong belief of being comfortable within your own skin and loving who you are will enhance your enjoyment of life and of your profession, leading you through difficult times.

Dan is Vice President of the American Society of Health-System Pharmacists (ASHP) Research and Education Foundation. Prior to ASHP, Dan had a distinguished practice as Director of the Finger Lakes Regional Poison and Drug Information Center and the Director of Emergency Medicine Research at the University of Rochester Medical Center in Rochester, New York. As Associate Director at the American Association of Poison Control Centers, he implemented the nationwide toll-free number for poison centers. He is also recognized as a Fellow of the American Academy of Clinical Toxicology, a Diplomat of the American Board of Applied Toxicology, and has served as President of the Association of Poison Control Centers of New York State.

He received his bachelor of science degree in pharmacy from the University of Pittsburgh and his doctor of pharmacy degree from Duquesne University. Dan completed a residency at Mercy Hospital of Pittsburgh and a clinical toxicology fellowship at the Pittsburgh Poison Center/Children's Hospital of Pittsburgh.

Any readers who have wondered about their ability to contribute or their "fit" in the profession will find value in Dan's message: *Love being exactly who you are.*

Dear Young Pharmacist,

To be effective in our professional roles as pharmacists, first we need to be comfortable in our own skin. This is something that I struggled with for decades. Many times over the last 30 years I have been asked, "When did you know that you were gay?" The reality is that I have always known. As early as the tender age of 6 years, I knew that I was different somehow. As a teenager, in the late 1970s, I began to struggle with coming to terms with being gay. As you can imagine, on some levels it was even harder then than it is today. Simply stated, the world was different and, to be honest, there was a lot more blatant discrimination in our society. There were no visible role models— family members, friends, political leaders, athletes, entertainers—who could provide a sense of normalcy to a confused adolescent.

Nonetheless, as I entered pharmacy school at the University of Pittsburgh in 1983, I began a 13-year journey of coming out. It was a scary time. In the spring of that year, AIDS made the covers of *Time* and *Newsweek*. I was a 20-year-old gay man who was beginning a difficult journey that was made harder by the weight of the AIDS epidemic. At that time, we did not know what microorganism caused the disease, how it was transmitted, or how to diagnose it. It was terrifying to think that a death sentence might be one of the implications of being the person that I was born to be. I heard disparaging comments about homosexuality from health professionals in the pharmacy school and in hospitals where I trained as we learned about and provided care to individuals with AIDS. During Professor Rounds one morning during my residency, the team went in to see a 30-something man, who was incarcerated at the time, admitted to the hospital for treatment of an AIDS-related infection. I remember the professor, an esteemed attending physician, harshly questioning the patient about the sexual activities that led to his HIV infection. At the time, I wondered if his approach to me would be equally judgmental if he knew that I was gay. The fear that I experienced made it impossible for me to be comfortable with myself; in retrospect, I realize that it affected both personal and professional relationships.

How much thought have you given to the relationship between who you are as a person versus who you are as a professional? Today, I clearly recognize that my ability to be effective in a professional role is directly connected to my comfort with being open about the person that I am. Throughout pharmacy school, a PharmD program, residency, and fellowship, I worked to ensure that my sexuality would never be known to "non-gay" people. I was afraid of losing family and friends and of discrimination at school and work. At the time, I did not realize how much of life—both personal and professional—I was missing by hiding. I also did not comprehend the connection between the personal and the professional. I know that there were friendships and professional opportunities lost because I would not allow people to get too close for fear that my secret would be revealed.

There was a direct relationship between my level of comfort with who I was and my ability to engage empathetically and compassionately with my patients. In addition, I believe that many of my professional successes are rooted in relationships, and these cannot be easily categorized as professional or personal. There is overlap, and often it is that personal connection that makes the difference. When I was hiding who I was, it was impossible to establish true relationships. Three people who are close friends and colleagues, Dr. Kim Coley, Dr. Edward Krenzelok, and Dean Patricia Kroboth, were part of my life during those times of fear. Kim, one of my oldest friends, was my lab partner in pharmacy school, Ed was my fellowship director, and Pat was my chairwoman when I was on the faculty at the University of Pittsburgh. Although each was incredibly supportive when I was hiding the real me, our relationships are so much deeper since I came out to them that I wish that I had done it sooner.

Some would argue that professional opportunities might have been lost if I had been open about my sexuality. To be frank, I probably would not have been as successful, or supported, in some of the faith-based institutions in which I worked. With the benefit of years of reflection and experience, I now realize that I would have found more inclusive environments that would have embraced me for the person and pharmacist that I was.

Two life events gave me the courage to become more public about who I was. First, I made the decision to move from my hometown of Pittsburgh to Rochester, New York. With that move to a new city, I decided to live my life without fear of people knowing that I was a gay man. My boss, Dr. Sandra Schneider, invited me to join the faculty as she became the chairwoman of the University of Rochester's Department of Emergency Medicine. I accepted on the condition that we have an important conversation. Her response was, "I know what it is and we only have to talk about it if you want to." This was the first time that I talked with a supervisor about my sexuality, and she put me at complete ease and helped make it possible to begin living openly as a gay man. My decision about openness was fortified by the second event—the loss of a dear friend, a wonderful 35-year-old dentist, to the AIDS epidemic. Steve's death put many things in perspective. These events also gave me the courage to begin conversations with my mother and sisters about my sexuality. Once I came out to my family, I had little fear of what others would think because the people who meant the most to me in life accepted me and reaffirmed their love. My ability to become comfortable in my own skin was key to entering into a loving relationship with my spouse, Nicolas.

The changes that we have witnessed in the first two decades of the 21st century have been dizzying. We have watched society change at a rapid pace, and numerous businesses and organizations of all sizes, including the American Society of Health-System Pharmacists (ASHP), have recognized that a person's sexuality does not affect his or her ability to do a job. I have also witnessed the effects of these societal changes in the profession of pharmacy. It is heartening to attend an ASHP meeting and encounter pharmacists whose same-sex partners or spouses accompany them to the meeting to share in the celebrations of their career successes. Such societal changes have helped me become increasingly more comfortable with who I am, and I hope that you, too, can draw strength from them. Yet, although we have seen amazing progress, you will need to evaluate professional opportunities in the context of your ability to live openly as the person you are. There are still areas in the United States where you may not have legal protections against workplace discrimination or workplace situations where you will not be completely supported because of missions and visions that are not supportive of gay people. Remember—If you allow discrimination to prevent you from being comfortable with who you are, it will negatively affect your ability to be successful in your professional role.

Our profession, with its reputation for being somewhat conservative in nature, presents its own challenges. I can only hope that my openness helps others become more comfortable with themselves. We must continue to develop a society where we treat sexual orientation, race, religion, ethnicity, and other differences the same as we treat eye color. As members of a caring profession, it is imperative that we embrace those who are different than we are and, hopefully, come to celebrate those differences.

What advice can I give to you? As I reflect on what I might have done differently over the last 30 years, I wish I had realized much sooner that it is okay to live as an openly gay man. A dear friend and mentor sent me a card for my birthday that said, *"Forever stay open, curious, fearless, transparent, and willing to be and love being exactly who you are."* While giving advice from a greeting card might seem trite, it is probably the best advice that I can give to you. I wish I had been honest earlier with people that I cared for as I could have shared so much more with them. I will never get those moments or that time back.

If you are struggling with who you are, I urge you to be open and honest. There will be difficult moments that will require courage as your family and friends process this new information, but I truly believe that those who love you will accept you for the person that you are. At that intersection of the personal and professional, achieving complete comfort with who you are as a person will enable you to be a better pharmacist and experience even greater career successes.

Sincerely,
*Daniel J. Cobaugh*

# Debra S. Devereaux

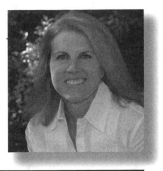

## *Life Is What Happens*
## *While You Are Busy Making Other Plans*

Deb Devereaux approached her career with a well-thought-out plan. She selected pharmacy as her career path because it would allow her the opportunity to build on her keen interest in science and the flexibility to raise a family while also pursuing a career. She spent summers working as an intern in various practice settings to determine which would be the best fit for her interests and methodically chose to pursue a business degree to help achieve her goals. Despite the meticulous planning, she readily admits that some other factors converged to influence her career path: personal relationships, her pharmacy colleagues and mentors, and serendipity. In the world of pharmacy, Deb's career has turned out to be somewhat unusual. Leveraging the skills she developed in hospital pharmacy management and through her MBA training, she has become one of the nation's experts on pharmacy reimbursement issues and the Medicare Part D benefit.

Deb is currently Senior Vice President of Pharmacy Services at Gorman Health Group. She received her bachelor of science degree in pharmacy from the University of Colorado and a master's degree in business administration from Regis University. She is a board certified ambulatory care pharmacist.

Deb's advice to young pharmacists is: *approach life with a plan and a strong dose of open mindedness and flexibility, seek out mentors, and help and support others.*

Dear Young Pharmacist,

I appreciate the opportunity to write to you regarding my pharmacy career, because I feel it is always good to reflect on how you got here and why you came. Perhaps some of the forks in my road will assist you in envisioning your own future.

I grew up in Western Colorado in a small picturesque mountain town. In high school, one of my after-school jobs was to wrap Christmas presents at the local pharmacy. The relief pharmacist, Theo Colburn, and I spoke about my interest in science and possible career choices. She encouraged me to look at pharmacy school because it was a great science career option, and you could easily combine it with raising a family. I enrolled at the University of Colorado and was accepted to pharmacy school. I specifically selected different intern opportunities (retail, industry, and hospitals) so I could decide where I felt I would be happiest. Although I liked the patient interactions at the retail pharmacy, I did not want to sell nail polish or make coke floats. I found the pharmaceutical manufacturer experience fascinating but missed seeing patients. I loved the hospital experience—exciting environment, bright and engaged colleagues, and interesting work. I was hired at the hospital after graduation and was promoted to supervisor and then assistant director after three years.

The years spent in the hospital were an excellent beginning for my career because it gave me the opportunities to work on committees and teams with physicians and nurses; build new clinical programs; get grounded in resource management and budgets, personnel management, and conflict resolution; and teach students, interns, technicians, and pharmacists. I was a voting member of the Institutional Review Board, which allowed me to have a front row seat into research projects and work with nursing and physician specialists. It became apparent to me that an advanced degree in business would be helpful in my career and conceivably be a requirement down the road. I originally intended to pursue a post baccalaureate doctor of pharmacy degree and residency but a marriage proposal and a husband with a Denver-based job tipped the balance. I began a traditional MBA program when my son was six months old and finished six months after my daughter was born—three-and-a-half years of classes two nights a week. It was difficult to juggle all my obligations, but I did it by assessing priorities every week. On those occasions when the babies were sick or some other disaster struck, I leaned on family and friends.

My mentor at the hospital was very active in the state hospital pharmacy association and encouraged me to become a member and volunteer for activities. I was elected to two different offices at the state level. He also took me to my first American Society of Health-System Pharmacists (ASHP) Midyear meeting, introduced me to other colleagues, and encouraged me to volunteer for a Special Interest Group advisory committee. I was hooked. I loved meeting colleagues from around the country, benefited tremendously from the shared information, and soaked up the continuing education. From my current Past President status to election to the Council on Administrative Affairs, and serving as state delegate, the experiences and the friends I have made have been incredible. It is true that the more time you give to professional organizations, the more you will get back in return.

A family move to a northern Colorado community necessitated a career change and the job I was originally slated to start did not materialize. Once again, my pharmacy colleague connections ensured that another door opened. I was recruited to begin the Drug Utilization Review program mandated by the federal legislation in OBRA 1990. The contract was with the School of Pharmacy so I was once again in an academic environment. I coordinated and facilitated a very active Pharmacy and Therapeutics Committee/DUR Board, and still found time to attend all the soccer games, ballet lessons, swim meets, and teacher conferences wearing my "mom hat."

I have now arrived at the third stop in my varied career journey. Because of my involvement in Medicaid, I was recruited to work in the Medicare Prescription Drug Program at its inception in 2006. We work with health plans and Pharmacy Benefit Management organizations to ensure compliance and to solve a myriad of operations and clinical issues. Every project is completely different, but the knowledge base is still basically the same. The goal is to ensure high quality access to medications and providers and deliver exceptional customer service to our clients. The work involves about 60 percent travel, which is sometimes frustrating and tiring, but the projects are challenging and never repetitive and the process of helping clients is very rewarding.

So, what wisdom do I have for you about your journey? I do know several things to be true:

- *Life is what happens while you are busy making other plans* (John Lennon).

  It is important to chart goals for your career. You do not want to just see how things unfold. It is also important to exist in your life "in the moment"—don't spend all your time looking back or looking forward. Enjoy the experiences you have and face up to the challenges presented. It may not be easy, but every experience teaches you something about yourself...unfortunately the negative experiences sometimes teach you the most.

- *Courage is being scared to death and saddling up anyway* (John Wayne).

  Jump at opportunities. Success is usually the result of some good luck and an awful lot of hard work. Waiting to be invited to participate or to be noticed that you are the right person for a promotion or a committee or a position will not make it happen. Plan to communicate. Practice an "elevator speech" about what makes you the right person for the opportunity.

- *It's what you learn after you know it all that counts* (John Wooden).

  Find the people who are best at what they do and ask them or allow them to mentor you. Mentors hold up the mirror and ask if this is what you want your life to look like. You need different mentors for different stages of your life. Find them, spend time with them, and ask for help when you are stuck.

- *Bloom where you are planted* (Saint Francis de Sales).

  Be serious about your commitments without being a serious person. Life is messy and funny. Laugh long and hard. No one has a perfect life, and spending your time being envious of other people's circumstances means that you are not living your own. Embrace the fact that every day is different from the day before. There are people and opportunities that will present themselves when you least expect them to.

- *The path to a truly successful and significant life is through friendship, through family, and through acts of generosity and self-sacrifice* (Rabbi Harold Kushner).

  You will refresh your own sense of purpose and your spirit by helping others. Give your colleagues the gifts of respect and acceptance. Give your friends and family the gifts of time and attention. You can never do enough for the people that you love and who love you. The relationships with the people you meet along the way are the lasting legacy of a purposeful life.

Finally, I will tell you that I feel that being a pharmacist is not my job, it is who I am; I think that the most successful and content pharmacists also feel the same way. Good luck!

Sincerely,
*Deb Devereaux*

# Sharon Murphy Enright

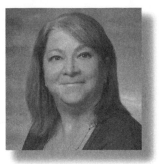

## *Lessons Learned from Others' Experiences Enrich Our Lives*

Sharon is an extremely creative, innovative, and entrepreneurial pharmacist. She continually reads literature outside of pharmacy and health care and has always thought deeply about where pharmacy needs to go and how she can assist practitioners. Sharon is great at making and seizing learning opportunities and has developed and conducted two startup education and training businesses—one of which she sold to a major corporation. She is a master at assisting people in applying business and nonpharmacy literature by developing and conducting educational programs for close to 100,000 pharmacists and other health care professionals. Sharon's recent involvement has focused on developing, implementing, and conducting the year-long online ASHP Foundation's Pharmacy Leadership Academy as well as authoring the Foundation's Leadership Resource Center. She is currently the Course Master and a primary faculty member for the ASHP Foundation's Pharmacy Leadership Academy and President of EnvisionChange LLC.

Sharon completed her bachelor of science in pharmacy degree at the University of Connecticut and a master's of administration, business, and behavioral sciences degree from George Washington University. She completed a residency at Yale–New Haven Hospital and Medical Center and the ASHP Executive Residency. Her letter indicates that since any knowledge has a very short and increasingly limited lifespan, it is only through continued growth and learning that we can continue to contribute. She ends her letter by saying, *love your work but don't make it your life.*

Dear Young Pharmacist,

The opportunity to gain from the sage advice of experienced leaders is an invaluable advantage in our hectic and complex world. Every lesson we learn from the experience of others will make your journey through life richer and more rewarding. The perspective provided by the experience of others creates a lens through which to view options, opportunities, and the directions our lives can offer.

My greatest and most memorable personal experience with early sage advice was unique. After finishing a residency at Yale–New Haven Hospital, I was fortunate to be selected as a Resident in the American Society of Health-System Pharmacists (ASHP) Executive Residency—a one-year training program in professional policy and association management. One of my first assignments was to staff the Residency Conference. Unbelievably, I found myself at dinner with Paul Parker, Cliff Latiolais, Don Francke, Don Brody, and Warren McConnell enjoying a part in a conversation about professional practice issues, goals, and aspirations, inviting me to be an active participant in the dialog. Their generous advice and interest set me on paths I could not have imagined before and gave me insights it would have taken decades to assimilate.

I have chosen to focus my advice to you on learning. During my ASHP-accredited residency at Yale, I was assigned a very wise mentor/preceptor—Gary McCart. One of our first conversations involved assessing my education and training and my confidence in my readiness for practice. Although I was successful academically and felt comfortable with the knowledge I had gained, I knew that I was not well enough prepared clinically to feel confident in independent practice. Gary helped me to recognize that deficiency as a gift, giving me the awareness and will to gain the clinical skills I would need *if* I chose clinical pharmacy as my career. More importantly, he helped me realize that most knowledge has a very short and increasingly limited lifespan and only through continued growth and learning could I contribute as a professional leader. My belief and commitment to continuous learning as a means to finding career options took root.

My second turning point occurred when I was the Director of Membership Services at ASHP. While at ASHP, a former professor and Executive Director of the American Association of Colleges of Pharmacy (AACP), Chris Rodowskas, would stop by and prod and encourage me to return to school. He made a committed and persistent investment in my learning and growth. Returning to school resulted in learning experiences that changed my life, my focus, and perspective and established a lifelong passion for systems thinking, knowledge and change management, and leadership. This exposure to new thinking and ideas formed in me a foundational belief that data-driven quality and performance improvement were the future of our profession and our health care systems. This is a path I might have missed without that persistent message to return to school, to keep learning, and to stretch and grow in new directions without limitation of traditional boundaries.

The following two thoughts are based on my personal experience. First, differentiate yourself in today's market place. A professional degree and license to practice will not be enough. With the growing numbers of students pursuing residency training and a more competitive market for leadership talent, you need every advantage to stand out from the crowd. Formalized leadership training (consider the Pharmacy Leadership Academy and other offerings available through ASHP and the ASHP Foundation) and an advanced degree (MBA, MHA, MPH, etc.) will not only hone your critical and strategic thinking, capabilities, and perspective, but will also allow you to provide unique and expanded value to your organization and other potential employers.

Second, actively explore ideas, literature, disciplines, and expertise beyond the strict boundaries of pharmacy, your specialty, and health care. You never know where your great ideas will come from, how seemingly disparate thoughts can come together for breakthrough knowledge, and the unique opportunities that far-afield learning may create. Think BIG, expand your focus, and enjoy learning for learning's sake.

Great leaders are defined by their commitment to their convictions. Knowing yourself and understanding the boundaries of your convictions are essential to standing by your principles, even when it costs you to do so. I have faced several critical moments in my career, facing alternatives (or directives) that just did not feel right and did not align with my belief and value system. The time spent thinking about my beliefs, professional values, and my vision for my role in the world, served as a ready baseline for making hard choices. There will be times and circumstances that are not subject to situational leadership. *A further word of advice:* it helps having a financial cushion to allow you the ability to stand on your principles. Without that cushion you may end up compromising in ways you never considered.

Learning—in fields and disciplines near and far to your focus—also provides you with perspective and a context for why and how your knowledge, skills, and talents are relevant in the larger world. Continuous learning enhances your capacity to make sense of the sometimes chaotic and overwhelming aspects of our increasingly complex human systems. Learning, testing your own convictions through dialog, reading, and self-reflection will help you to find your passion for your life's work, your voice for leading others, and your commitment to work hard to achieve your goals. You will never know when or how your convictions and values might be tested. But without the knowledge gained from your experience and the experience of others, you will be ill-prepared to react, to lead, and to transform yourself so you can survive and thrive.

How to use information effectively for ourselves and our organizations is another challenge you will face. There is no shortage of information in our world. In fact, it can be overpowering. As *The New York Times* columnist Thomas Friedman states, each of us needs to bring new *value to our work* every day, above and beyond the job we were hired to do. As quality and safety experts Batalden and Davidoff state, we must go to work each day with two jobs in mind—the one we were hired to do as well as improving the job we were hired to do. You must constantly refresh your knowledge pool.

I think the best learning occurs not in isolation but with others in dialog, discussion, debate, and sharing of our knowledge. Our world is changing fast. Only those with the ability to learn collaboratively will have the creativity and foresight to protect themselves from being blinded by what we think we know with certainty. Sharing what we know, think, and observe gives us the joy of those "aha" moments, the exhilarating breakthroughs, and the excitement of discovery.

Life and career transformations have been the norm, not the exception, in my career. For you, have an awareness of your environment and anticipate change. Have the ability to piece together disparate ideas in a way that makes sense of the often crazy paradoxes you will face. Most importantly, maintain strong networks of trusted professional relationships to give yourself access to needed insight and perspective. I recommend reading *The Power of Flow: Transforming Your Life with Meaningful Coincidence* (Belitz and Lundstrom, Harmony Press, 1998).

Live a happy life. Cherish the changes that come your way. Love your work but don't make it your life.

Best,
*Sharon Murphy Enright*

# Jeanne Rucker Ezell

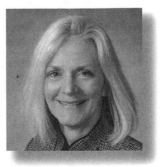

## *Building Relationships Is an Essential Part of Leadership*

Jeanne's friends and colleagues know her as a dedicated person focused on her family, profession, and her goals. She always has a vision and a plan, and she knows how to execute. Execution to Jeanne is not only about getting it done, but getting it done the right way. She always has the "greater good" in mind when she executes a plan. Just as important, everyone knows that she cares about what she does.

Jeanne's educational background and training certainly prepared her well for her leadership roles. She received her bachelor of science degree from the University of Tennessee College of Pharmacy, and her master of science degree and residency from the University of Kansas. She is currently the Director of Pharmacy and Residency Program at Blount Memorial Hospital in Maryville, Tennessee. Jeanne is not only a leader in health-system pharmacy practice, but also in her community as she consistently serves in volunteer leader positions.

During her career, she has understood and valued the importance of relationships in accomplishing goals, building productive cultures, and job satisfaction. She is very clear in her message that *leadership is required for successful and sustained change and that relationships that demonstrate genuine dedication and caring are an essential part of leadership.*

Dear Young Pharmacist,

I believe all pharmacists must be leaders. You do not have to be in a formal leadership role to be a leader in our profession. No matter where you work or your position, our profession needs you to be a good leader. After 25 years as a hospital pharmacy director, I find every day I am still striving to become a better leader. I share my experience in hopes that it will benefit you as a leader in your workplace.

I come from a family of hard workers, and if you were to ask any of the people I have worked with, I think they would describe me as a hard worker as well. But after more than 30 years in the pharmacy profession, I prefer to be known for the impact I may have had on people's lives rather than the fact that I worked really hard! I love that my parents instilled in me the notion that I could accomplish anything I desired if I worked hard. But in addition to hard work it takes leadership to develop a strong pharmacy service. No matter what your position, we all have important responsibilities in this profession, and how we carry them out is what really makes a difference in people's lives.

In my early days as a pharmacy director, I prided myself on good organizational and strategic planning skills, setting goals and accomplishing them, and always treating my staff fairly. I participated in Stephen Covey's Seven Habits of Highly Effective People training program and have really tried to incorporate those seven habits into my life. In 1990, I took a second director of pharmacy position with the challenge of expanding and improving pharmacy services. One of the pharmacists did medication use reviews and nursing education and another pharmacist provided medication education for cardiac rehabilitation patients, but the pharmacy did not provide any other clinical services. The nursing director was eager to implement computerized medication administration records and a complete intravenous admixture service. However, I encountered little enthusiasm for change from many of my pharmacy staff. A few people were excited about making improvements, but there were also some vocal staff who asked, "Why should we do that to help the nurses?" After that, I added *culture change* to my *needs improving* list. I soon realized that working hard planning and implementing changes was not the answer unless I could personally lead a majority of the staff in the desire for change.

I learned that part of leadership is using all the tools available to you. I engaged our hospital's employee assistance program to help improve teamwork among the pharmacy staff so that we could utilize small planning groups to become more effective in carrying out new goals and objectives. A tool used by the employee assistance program was the Myers Briggs Personality Test followed with individual and group sessions with a counselor. I was reminded that each individual is different, learns and interacts with others in a preferred style, and I should approach each person as an individual. For example, some of my staff needed to be slowly introduced to a change to let them contemplate the potential impact and formulate questions and reactions to the change. Others might be so excited about the change; they would be ready to jump right in and start planning right away. This experience with Myers Briggs testing reminded me to think more about each person on my staff as an individual and in terms of their personal preferences.

At that point in time, my staff was small enough for me to know each person, and I had met most of their families at pharmacy social events. I very much enjoyed this interaction and the relationship with my staff. As my staff grew, it became harder to really get to know each individual beyond their work identity. For some employees, there were few opportunities to talk socially; for others, such as our pharmacy practice residents, there were multiple opportunities. I was afraid losing touch with some on my staff would become a problem, and, of course, my fear was realized. I had a rude awakening a couple of years ago, when a disgruntled technician told me, "You are the coldest boss I have ever had, and you don't care anything about the pharmacy staff." Even though I knew this technician was angry because of a disciplinary action for violation of a work policy, her comments stung and gave me pause to reflect that perhaps some of my staff did not know that I cared about them. We know all too well that the answer to the question, "Do you commit to a leader that does not care about you?" is very clear: *No*.

On self examination, I realized that the majority of my interactions with staff members were almost 100% about work. Even though I intentionally worked a variety of hours to ensure I was accessible to all shifts throughout the week, I tried to conserve their time and mine by discussing mostly work-related issues. Near the time of this personal awakening, I read Disney executive Lee Cockerell's book, *Creating Magic: 10 Common Sense Leadership Strategies from a Life at Disney*. What impressed me the most about his story was how obviously important his personal attentiveness to his associates was to Disney's success.

Because I really do care about each of them, I decided that I would interact with at least one of my staff every day on a more personal level, inquiring about their weekend, their sick parent, or their child's ballgame, for example. After all, I spend more waking hours with my pharmacy family than I do my own. It has taken some effort to make sure I find a good time each day to specifically reach out on a personal level to one of my staff who I might not otherwise have an opportunity to see or speak with. I found that I enjoy taking time each day to talk with staff members about a topic that has nothing to do with work, and I see most are quite happy to share a little of what's important to them. Today we have a department with a culture of continuous improvement and an ongoing objective of building a strong pharmacy service. Everyone knows their role and understands the importance of their role in making a difference in people's lives.

As you move forward in your career, I encourage you to take time to get to know the people with whom you work, other pharmacists, and health care providers. The connections I have made with nurses, physicians, students, residents, patients, and others I have encountered are what I find most enjoyable.

Never get so busy that you feel a few minutes connecting with a fellow employee is wasteful. Those personal connections are key to your success as a work team, and can bring more joy and understanding into everyone's work day. Some of my best work memories are of staff members who have grown into outstanding pharmacists or technicians, and I consider it an honor to know them.

Do not forget that you are a leader and improving pharmacy services requires leadership.

My wish for you is that you can use my advice to help you be a more effective leader in your workplace and in our great profession!

Sincerely,
*Jeanne Ezell*

# Kate Farthing

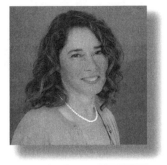

## *Knowing Yourself*

On meeting Kate you will quickly conclude that she is a person who is passionate about learning. She also is passionate about her role as a preceptor and training pharmacy residents in drug information and drug policy skills. Finally, you will find that Kate is a person of high integrity, possesses vast clinical knowledge, and maximizes that knowledge in drug and practice policy decisions. These are all characteristics that have contributed to her success in clinical practice and drug policy development.

Currently, Kate practices as a clinical pharmacy specialist with responsibilities for quality and patient safety at Legacy Health in Portland, Oregon. Previously, she practiced at Oregon Health and Sciences University Hospitals and Clinics in drug information and drug policy and as the Director of the Drug Information Specialty Residency Program and PGY1 residency program director. She is also active in state and national pharmacy organizations.

Kate received her doctor of pharmacy degree from the University of Kansas and completed a specialty residency in drug information at the University of Kansas Medical Center. In the spirit of life-long learning, she completed the American Society of Health-System Pharmacists Foundation Pharmacy Leadership Academy Program and now serves as one of its faculty members. Among her passions are training and mentoring pharmacy residents and others at the early stages of their career. Thus it is not surprising that her message in the following letter reflects on wisdom gained during her residency training: *Knowing yourself and how you need to prepare are critical to your performance especially in anxiety creating situations.*

Dear Young Pharmacist,

T his is a moment in time (well, several moments) that we really do need to explore. The event haunts you, and we have learned much about ourselves moving forward. Through a series of conflicts and scheduling problems, the first Pharmacy and Therapeutics Committee meeting of your drug information specialty residency was five months into the program. The agenda was packed, and you worked hard to verify the accuracy of the meeting packets— each of the eight formulary requests were printed on a different color of paper, the reports were ready, and the other residents presenting items were prepared for the meeting. The director of pharmacy and drug information service director were on edge that afternoon; there was too much material to reasonably cover in the 90-minute meeting and two of the items were controversial, with strong-willed physicians in attendance. You presented the third formulary request, a unique antipsychotic drug with solid clinical trials and a relatively clean safety profile, according to the monograph prepared by a student you precepted in the drug information service three months ago. The agenda pace was brisk, and it was your turn to introduce the next formulary request. No words emerged from your mouth, your mind was completely blank as you felt all eyes in the room rise up from the monograph printed on goldenrod-colored paper and stare at you.

There was still nothing from you and the silence became uncomfortable as you felt the heat in the room and your blood pressure rise. The drug information director stated your name as a second introduction, and still your mind was blank. The tension was palpable, and the director prompted, "Tell us about the new antipsychotic drug Dr. Wilson requested." Luckily, this jarred you back to the present moment, and words began tumbling from your mouth. To this day, you cannot recall what exactly was said by you or about the drug, but the meeting finally ended, and the discussion around the awkward start began (and remains forever etched in your mind).

Being nervous is expected and managing nervousness becomes easier over time with a few strategies that will serve you well— be organized, be on time, and be prepared. Over the next 20 years, the struggle with those first words continues in many situations; professional presentations are the most obvious, but speaking up in a free-flowing conversation is frequently uncomfortable, too. The article, "Using Self-Talk to Enhance Career Satisfaction and Performance"[*] offers valuable advice that gives us the tools to master the concept of self-talk by encouraging us to open up and share an idea that may not be thoroughly formulated during a conversation. It advises us to learn a few easy-to-use motivating phrases that really help as you go into a meeting or join a group already deep in discussion.

My father gave me some of the best advice after that awkward silence of the Pharmacy and Therapeutics Committee meeting—you need to know more than most in the room. In hindsight, the monograph prepared by another learner in the chaos leading up to a busy meeting was my downfall. I needed to embrace the assigned content and make the details of the request my own, rather than attempting to rephrase the work of another. Fortunately, I picked up this learning quickly. Now, I own the material and commit to memory the first statement to start the presentation or conversation. These successful techniques carried me through residency and my early career.

Today, the advice I give you is to invest in yourself by learning who you are and how you are programmed to operate.

- Get to know your personality and behaviors—use an accessible personality assessment such as the DiSC behavioral style or Myers Briggs Type Indicator (MBTI).

- Take the time to explore what the evaluation means both professionally and personally.

- Understand how you take in, share, and process technical information as well as information necessary to make decisions.

Understanding your personality, how you work with others, and how others perceive or react to you will be an invaluable asset to help build confidence and lead yourself through the exciting years ahead.

Take a deep breath and appreciate the opportunities presented each day—it's going to be a great career!

Take care,
*Kate*

---

[*]White SJ. Using self-talk to enhance career satisfaction and performance. *Am J Health-Syst Pharm.* 2008; 65(6):514-519.

# Joyce A. Generali

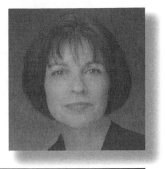

*Don't Fret about Career and Personal Life*
*Balance—There Is No Such Thing*

As you meet Joyce it is immediately obvious she is a gregarious extrovert who has a great sense of humor, and with little prompting she will tell you a joke, many on herself. It is thus easy to imagine her early experience as a bus tour guide telling jokes to keep her charges engaged. Joyce has a serious side as she is an expert and proficient drug information specialist. She put together all the Black Box warnings and published them thus alerting and enabling practitioners to protect patients. Joyce brings a number of years of experience in conducting drug information centers and teaching as a pharmacy faculty while raising a family.

Joyce holds a bachelor of science in pharmacy from the University of Connecticut, School of Pharmacy and a master of science degree from The University of Kansas, School of Pharmacy. She completed residencies at the Medical College of Virginia Hospitals and Kansas University Medical Center. Joyce is currently Director, Synthesized Referential Content, Facts and Comparisons and Professor Emeritus, Kansas University School of Pharmacy.

In her letter, she gives the following advice: *Saying goodbye to "perfect" and hello to "it's done" and learning the difference between the two is a key to being comfortable with the decisions you make on how to spend your time.*

Dear Young Pharmacist,

D on't fret so much about *balance*. The eternal quest, or should I say struggle, for the how to live a productive personal AND work life is a question for the ages. There is no balance. Sometimes it is 60/40; sometimes it is 80/20. Sometimes, it feels fine to be 30/70, and other times you feel totally out of whack at 55/45. Here's why. Balance is an imperfect concept. It is a static term, a snapshot of time attempting to define a dynamic process. It is a moving target. Each day it feels different. A set of changing probabilities and possibilities that looks one way before your morning cup of coffee and another way on the way driving home from work. Balance is a myth that we all chase, something just out of reach, right around the corner. If we just stretched a little harder, we would have it. Right?

Stop chasing the shadow and look up to see what is really in front of you. Imbalance only rears its head when we feel out of control. At its core, the yearning for balance is really about our expectations and the strong desire to do all things well. Not having balance is just another way to describe that we are stressed.

I never expected balance in my residency programs. I knew what I signed up for. But once I was in the work world on my own, I did expect some sort of settling down. And it never happened. For me, it was raising a family while working full time without family close by. For you, it might be a different set of expectations for the lines between your professional and personal world. It might be growing personal responsibilities: caring for elderly parents, merging schedules with a spouse, or finding enough time to train for a marathon during a particularly busy time at work. Handling stress and making thoughtful decisions about priorities in both life and work are the keystones to being and feeling productive.

I remember an important decision point in my career, one which forced me to reprioritize my goals in a more responsible and accountable way, and ultimately reduce the imbalance or stress that I was feeling. I was about 10 years into a solid career and was working full time, married to a partner with a very busy career, and had two children. I was responsible for the vast majority of the domestic tasks. At this very busy time, I was appointed to a national council for a professional organization. I had successfully served on national committees before and did not anticipate a problem. Accepting the appointment meant that I was committing myself toward a leadership path in a very specific area on a national level. It was in an area that was not part of my main career goals, but it was a great opportunity and some of my favorite colleagues were involved. One year into a three-year commitment, I was overwhelmed on several levels. The travel was significant, I was behind in everything, and I did not feel that I was doing anything well, at work or at home. At first, I was stubborn. In past similar scenarios, I just worked harder. But putting my nose to the grindstone was not going to help in this case. It took another two months to realize that I made a mistake. It felt like a failure—and a big one at that. But after a long and deep reflective assessment, I realized that my participation on this particular panel, although beneficial, was not really in my core career goals. There were only so many hours in the day. I resigned. Immediately, a weight was lifted from my shoulders. It was a difficult and painful decision; however, through it, I learned that I could prioritize my activities that allowed for reality-based productivity. Nearly 20 years later, I look back and realize that it was a turning point. Successes have come in other areas and in a less stressful environment.

Regardless of the specific causes, life is uneven. There will be times—absolutely guaranteed—when you do not feel like you are doing anything well, or only doing some things well and not the ones that are most important to you. Say goodbye to "perfect" and say hello to "it's done" and learn the difference between the two. Now that I look back on those moments of imbalance, this is what I see. I see a stretching of personal resources and development of patience and compassion. I see it as exactly the time that I learned to say *no* to opportunities that distracted from my main goals. Just because I could do something, did not mean I should.

I learned to:

- breathe in the moment,
- make hard choices,
- ask for help when it was needed,

- reassess in practical and responsible ways,
- know when to change paths, and
- do my best in the face of change.

Remember—stop looking at the scales and follow your internal compass. It will be fine.

*Joyce Generali*

# Lisa M. Gersema

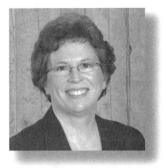

## *Most Rewarding Relationships with Physicians Require Hard Work*

After practicing as a clinical pharmacist and clinical pharmacy manager for the first 17 years of her career, Lisa changed courses; she became the Director of Pharmacy at United Hospital in St. Paul, Minnesota. In her letter, Lisa candidly reflects on some of the difficulties she experienced early in her career establishing peer relationships with other members of the health care team. She overcame those challenges by proving herself, doing her homework, and holding steadfast to her patient care recommendations, even when faced with skepticism, condescension, and just plain bad behavior. Lisa has observed how the profession has evolved since her early days of practice, making confrontations like those she experienced much less common for pharmacists entering practice now. She and other qualified clinical experts among our profession helped pave the way for this evolution and advance the role of pharmacists as highly skilled members of the patient care team. Lisa is committed to a career of continuous professional development and sharpening her skills, as evidenced by her completion of a master's in health care administration 27 years after completing her doctor of pharmacy degree.

Lisa is currently Director of Pharmacy and Residency Program Director at United Hospital in St. Paul, Minnesota. She received her bachelor of science and doctor of pharmacy degrees from the University of Iowa School of Pharmacy. She has served American Society of Health-System Pharmacists as chair of the Council on Pharmacy Practice, member of the Commission on Therapeutics, delegate to the House of Delegates, and a member of the board of directors. Lisa's message is: *With clinical decisions, it is important to present the evidence and then it becomes your job to sell it—both are critical skills to be successful as a pharmacist.*

Dear Young Pharmacist,

I can only imagine the changes that you will observe during your career. The practice of pharmacy has advanced significantly since I graduated. Today, we are much closer to the patients and collaborate with our nursing and physician colleagues on a regular basis. The value and purpose of a team approach is integrated into curriculums. Nurses, physicians, and others expect the pharmacist to be present on the patient care unit, to participate in rounds, and to contribute to patient care. It was not always that way.

When I began my career, physicians often scoffed at my recommendations and said that they would listen to me only after I had obtained my *medical* degree. Another approach of physicians was to not accept my recommendation when speaking to me in person. I would later discover, however, that the medication order was changed exactly to my recommendation. (I considered this saving-face maneuver a small victory!) I am pleased that these scenarios do not occur as often as they once did. I have counseled more than one student, resident, or young pharmacist through a difficult physician interaction involving inappropriate physician behavior that needed to be addressed. Others, however, involved reasonable questions that were expressed a bit sharper than the young pharmacist was accustomed to hearing. For those, I would often share one or both of the following experiences.

After completing my pharmacy training and fellowship, I sought employment at a hospital where I could help establish clinical pharmacy services. I was attracted to St. Luke's Hospital in Kansas City because they were hiring pharmacists with PharmDs to enhance their clinical pharmacy focus. At that time, gentamicin was a commonly prescribed antibiotic, and physicians routinely prescribed a standard 80 mg q8 regimen regardless of a patient's age, weight, renal function, site of infection, etc. Clearly, this was an opportunity for clinical pharmacy services! The Pharmacy Clinical Coordinator along with another PharmD pharmacist monitored all aminoglycoside patients when I started working at the hospital. This was the type of involvement and program building that I had hoped to find in my first pharmacist job. I was able to quickly jump in to assist with this coverage. Our goal was to have all pharmacists competent to evaluate the patient's pharmacokinetic profile and make recommendations appropriate for the infection. I worked with the staff individually to understand the rationale behind the equations and the impact of renal function, body size, age, etc. It was important to me that everyone understood the "why" as well as the "how." I took a great deal of ownership for this program and was very proud to see how the staff had responded. It was wonderful to watch the excitement demonstrated by pharmacists when gentamicin levels returned almost exactly as they had predicted and the patient was improving. This program was serving as our launching pad for more clinical services. Even after 25 years, I still feel a great sense of pride as I recall these memories.

So you can imagine my dismay when a senior surgical resident relayed his dislike of our aminoglycoside service to me during a casual conversation. The look on my face was likely one of utter shock! I asked him why he felt this way. His response gave me pause. He valued the pharmacist's role and usually accepted their recommendations. Occasionally, however, he would reject the recommendation to test the pharmacist's commitment to it. Too often, the pharmacist's response had simply been, "OK." If the pharmacist did not discuss the rationale with him, he questioned the recommendation's necessity or validity. I was never sure how many times this had occurred, but I certainly learned something that day. From that day forward, I worked with the staff to anticipate push back and to be prepared for it.

I personally experienced this type of "testing" from a cardiologist while rounding with the cardiology teaching service. The attending physicians who led the rounding teams rotated weekly. It gave me the opportunity to work with many cardiologists—each with their own personality and perspective. I enjoyed working with most of them. One, however, was especially difficult. He was a respected physician, had developed a large and well-respected private cardiology practice, was well connected in the community, and was arrogant and opinionated. I had heard stories how he intimidated medical residents, and he often rudely challenged me or criticized our department during rounds. I worked hard to stand tall against this—I remember clasping my hands behind my back during rounds so he could not see them shaking! When opportunities arose, I provided evidenced-based recommendations to improve a medication regimen. He sometimes accepted my recommendations; sometimes not.

One day, he called me to evaluate a patient who was not on the teaching service, who was a long-time patient of his, and the father of a colleague (in other words, a special patient!). The patient had a long list of medications, and the cardiologist was perplexed as to what was wrong with the patient. After my assessment, I suspected digoxin toxicity. I told the cardiologist and recommended ordering a digoxin level. His initial response was, "No, that can't be it, I just checked a digoxin level last week, and it was fine." I provided all of the rationale behind my decision. When this did not work, I finally said, "It smells like digoxin toxicity, just humor me and get a level." Somewhat to my surprise, he obliged and ordered one. Later that afternoon, the level returned, and it was greater than 4 ng/mL. I went to the patient care unit to discuss next steps with the physician and found that he had already reviewed the digoxin level. As I approached, he turned to his nurse clinician and said, "Deb, have you met Dr. Gersema?" Because I had worked with his nurse for several years, we both responded with a puzzled "yes." As I walked back to my office, it struck me what had just happened—his acknowledgment of me as "Doctor" Gersema was his way of saying that he finally recognized me as a trusted and valued colleague.

After that day, it was not unusual for him to call me to discuss medication-related concerns for patients that he was seeing in his office or in the hospital. I was told that even after I left this hospital, he inquired about me. As I reflect back on those early years, I realize that some of my most rewarding relationships with physicians may have been the ones that I had to work the hardest to obtain.

I am now a Director of Pharmacy. Many of the skills learned during those days as a clinical specialist are directly transferrable to my work today. I must confess, however, that I am still gaining insight regarding how much I should push when communicating with administrators or other leaders outside of pharmacy. Just as with clinical decisions, I must present the evidence, then I must sell it. Both of these are critical skills to be successful as a pharmacist. One without the other may work for some situations, but will not create a trusted and respected relationship with pharmacy or nonpharmacy colleagues.

Best wishes on your professional journey,
*Lisa Gersema*

# Diane B. Ginsburg

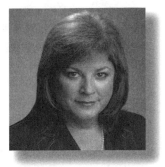

## Serve Your "Every Patient"

Those of us who know Diane well might describe her as someone unfazed by the level of stress that would send some right to the cardiologist, easily juggling priorities that would cause many to crack, and doing so in this season's premier designer shoes. When things start to feel manageable, Diane purposely goes in search of new challenges. As an example, she decided to pursue her doctorate degree at one of the busiest times of her life, a decision prompted by tragedy. Teaching is her passion, and she realized the degree would help her be a better professor and administrator. She finished her PhD coursework at the University of Texas at Austin with a perfect 4.0, of course.

Pharmacy was not in Diane's original career plans, but serendipity played a significant role in her career path. As with other aspects of Diane's life, once she decided to be a pharmacist she was all in, working almost full-time as a pharmacy intern while in pharmacy school.

Diane is currently Assistant Dean for Student Affairs and Clinical Professor of Health Outcomes and Pharmacy Practice at the University of Texas College of Pharmacy. She completed her bachelor of science degree in pharmacy at the University of Pittsburgh School of Pharmacy, a master of science degree in hospital pharmacy at the University of Houston College of Pharmacy, and completed a two-year ASHP-accredited residency in hospital pharmacy administration at The Methodist Hospital in Houston, Texas. An active American Society of Health-System Pharmacists (ASHP) member and volunteer, Diane is a past-president of ASHP and former chair of the board of the ASHP Research and Education Foundation.

Diane's letter describes *the concept of "every patient" taught to her by her mother*, a philosophy that has made her a better pharmacist.

Dear Young Pharmacist,

I did not start out wanting to be a pharmacist. I graduated high school a year early and went away to college right after I turned 17. I thought I wanted to be a surgeon like my uncle, who was chief of surgery at the University of Pittsburgh School of Medicine. I remember how he cared for his patients and talked to me about medicine. I was a good student in math, chemistry, and biology. Medicine was a good place for me. When I told my chemistry professor that I was pre-med, she suggested pharmacy school, as the curriculum was a great foundation for medical school. I remember telling the admissions committee that I had always wanted to be a pharmacist, that I had actually counted jellybeans with my mom's icing knife as preparation to fill prescriptions. I was lying through my teeth, as I had no idea what a pharmacist did. By some miracle, I was accepted. In 2005, I received the Distinguished Alumnus Award from the University of Pittsburgh School of Pharmacy. During my lecture to the students, I confessed and told them my story. My point in "coming clean" was that you never know where a path will lead you and to be open-minded. Had I not applied to pharmacy school, the wonderful opportunities that have come my way would have never been presented to me had I chosen a different direction.

In my first year in pharmacy school I learned the important lesson about "every patient" from my mother. My uncle had a very large surgical practice and needed someone to manage his office. He asked my mother, an accountant, to come and work for him. I watched how my uncle and mother cared for his patients. My mother would always tell me that every patient had a story; every patient was significant to someone. The patients were spouses, parents, grandparents, sisters and brothers, children, and friends. She would greet them with a smile, ask how they were doing, and listen to their answers. I was amazed how she did this with such sick people. What she told me stayed with me and guides my every decision:

*Remember, every patient is someone significant. When you care for your patients, most of them will be perfect strangers. These patients deserve the very best we have to give them;*

*we should use all of our resources, our knowledge to help them. Someday, someone significant to you might need care and hopefully their practitioners will treat your someone significant as if they were family. Always remember the significance of "every patient."*

In my final year of pharmacy school, I received an application from The Methodist Hospital in Houston, Texas. I accepted my father's dare, sent the application in, and received an interview. After meeting the hospital staff, I decided to see if I could move someplace where I did not know anyone and make it. I packed up my little yellow Ford Fiesta named Woodstock and moved to Houston.

I had to see if I could take everything I had learned and do what I had set out to do. I was scared and excited simultaneously. I am amazed I had the insight at 22 years of age to be confident in myself, and my abilities. I would hear my mother's voice in my head, "no matter how crazy your day is and/or what challenges you may be having, remember who your patients are and that their issues are far greater than yours."

The move to Houston truly changed the course of my life. During my first year of practice, I had the privilege to work with some amazing practitioners and mentors. The administrative team at Methodist and faculty at the University of Houston convinced me to enter their master of science in hospital pharmacy and joint residency program. I would be Methodist's first resident and the program would be submitted for the American Society of Health-System Pharmacists' (ASHP) accreditation following the completion of my two-year program. Had it not been for my graduate program, I would never have had the opportunity to teach and be exposed to academic pharmacy. The students I taught and supervised during rotations learned about my true north, my mother's concept of "every patient."

I thought I would practice in hospitals throughout my career until I gave a few guest lectures at the University of Texas at Austin College of Pharmacy. After meeting with faculty and the Dean, something inside me said to give this aspect of practice a try. I voiced my concern to my mother about giving up my patient care role. She said that I would have one degree of separation from patients. My students would be providing care for "every patient." She told me to trust my gut and heart, and I moved to Austin and started my life as an academic pharmacist.

In my new student orientations about professionalism, I made sure they understood about providing care for "every patient." I never thought that my words and teachings would come back to help me and my "every patient."

My mother decided she was going to retire and moved to Austin to be near me. She flunked retirement and was hired by the City of Austin to work with their clinics. Unfortunately, the time she had in Austin was very brief. My mother was diagnosed with pancreatic cancer. When we got the diagnosis, it was like an out-of-body experience. As a pharmacist when you hear this kind of diagnostic language, you immediately go into your clinical/problem-solving mode. Once that passes and you realize it is your family member, your reaction is completely different. Your clinical knowledge is your protection from the horrific events that are happening. As you can imagine, I was pretty distraught and tried to keep it together for my mother and my family. My mother's tumors made it very difficult to manage her pain. One of my former students, a newly licensed pharmacist, said, "We figured out how to manage your mother's pain, Diane. Don't worry; she is going to get some relief. I am going to take care of her."

I looked up at this young practitioner and asked, "Why are you being so kind to us?" He replied very simply, "All I am doing is what you told me to do that very first day of pharmacy school. Your mother is my 'every patient.'" I remember thinking in that moment that it would never matter what I did for the remainder of my professional life. I got through to one student who took care of my "every patient."

I have been fortunate to work with amazing people, serve the profession, and teach wonderful students. My compass is always with me—my mother's teachings. I hope my story and experience help you as you begin this phase of your professional and personal journey. Make the most of every experience and give of yourself to your profession and community. Some of you will serve your profession in a leadership position. Step up and accept the opportunity. Never forget why you entered this revered profession; our calling is to serve our patients. Always remember your "every patient" and give the very best you can in your care. I wish you all the best and look forward to seeing the mark your generation will make on this profession.

Warmest personal regards,
*Diane B. Ginsburg*

# Harold N. Godwin

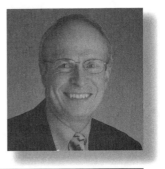

*Be Active and Shape Your Future
and Those Following in Your Path*

Harold is so passionate about pharmacy that in addition to his almost 50 years in practice, teaching, and academic leadership, he has continually given his personal time to professional organizations as well as residency training and teaching pharmacy students. What is remarkable about Harold is that he has always been able to step back and view issues from the perspective of the whole profession not just as a hospital/health-system pharmacist. He has rarely missed a national or state professional meeting, continues to be an instrumental part of whatever change is occurring (preferring not to be a victim), and continues to seize opportunities. His professional commitment is evidenced by his serving as president of the American Society of Health-System Pharmacists (ASHP), the American Council of Pharmacy Education (now known as the Accreditation Council for Pharmacy Education [ACPE]), and the American Pharmacists Association (APhA). In his 1991 Harvey AK Whitney Award Lecture, he outlined the converging paths leading to the development of pharmaceutical care, which moves pharmacists into direct patient care.

Harold received his bachelor of science in pharmacy degree at the University of Kansas and his master of science degree from The Ohio State University. He completed a residency at The Ohio State University Hospitals. He is currently Professor and Associate Dean of Pharmacy for Clinical and Medical Center Affairs at the University of Kansas, School of Pharmacy.

Harold ends his letter with excellent advice: *a successful career is not a destination, but it is the journey to success that is so very rewarding.*

Dear Young Pharmacist,

It gives me pleasure to write to you and provide some advice about achieving success in our great profession. Although I have had many outstanding mentors, I wish that someone would have provided me with cogent advice early in my career to focus my attention on becoming a more effective leader. You have a wonderful and exciting career ahead of you. Pharmacists today are in a dynamic profession that is poised for greatness. In your career you may assume roles not yet even imagined. Looking back on my career, here are some development and leadership tips that I wished I had known.

First, always be curious about both your profession and your colleagues. Soon you will find yourself in an interprofessional environment practicing in teams or organizations and not as an individual. The profession's success will be measured not only by our clinical and leadership abilities but by our interactions and relationships with the comprehensive team of different disciplines. You will be working side by side with other health care providers, managers, faculty, business professionals, patients, and the public at large. The better you understand your colleagues' career directions/goals and their aspirations, the more successful you will be in your career. Understand what makes your colleagues tick and understand your "big picture" environment. Health care reform is here, and changes in our profession will accelerate like never before. You should be an instrumental part of this transformation and not a victim of this change.

Second, capitalize on your strengths. As you continue to develop and grow in your career, you will realize that you have certain strengths as well as some weaknesses or areas that need improvement. Certainly, you should strive to improve those weak areas, but actually you should play to your own strengths. Demonstrate what you are good at and how you excel around others. An enlightening book is *Strengths Finder 2.0* by Tom Rath (Gallup Press). I encourage you to read it. This leadership text helps you identify your strengths and assists you in capitalizing on the value you have. It is also an excellent book for group study in your work environment. We need all strengths to be represented on any successful cohesive team.

Third, know when opportunity knocks. Throughout your career, you will have unexpected opportunities. And while these opportunities may be unexpected, always fully consider all paths presented. Some paths may take your career on a new and rewarding course. In my early career as a pharmacy department manager, I never thought I would be involved as an educator. As a new Assistant Director, I was assigned (really could not refuse) to teach a pharmacy course when a faculty member went on a sabbatical leave. I accepted this unexpected and unplanned opportunity. I found that I actually liked teaching. Consequently, I have been both an administrator and educator ever since. Often new opportunities become a catalyst to the success in your career. From a leadership standpoint, you may have an idea or a program that you feel should be implemented. However, you might find the opportunity or the timing is just not right. The key to success is knowing when an opportunity is at its peak for implementation. Many good ideas have been purposefully held back for just the right time. On the other hand, when the timing is right, move forward. Remember, sometimes it is better to ask forgiveness than permission.

Fourth, become actively involved in promoting and advancing your profession. To be a pharmacist is rewarding, and yet it demands a collective responsibility from all members to sustain and grow the profession. I have had a very rewarding career by being engaged in our profession through pharmacy organizations at the local, state, and national level. You should be an active member in our professional organizations. Start by volunteering for association committees. From there you can move to various elected offices and then, you never know—you may become a national officer as I have. My involvement in national leadership activities started with my volunteering to serve on a pharmacy organization committee.

You have already gained much from the pharmacy profession. Now it is your responsibility to give back by engaging in the profession's activities to create an even better profession for your future pharmacy colleagues. Do not opt to sit on the sidelines and let your colleagues shape the profession for you. Be active and shape not only your future but the future of those following in your path.

Fifth, network, network, network. Pharmacy is a small world, but it is created by being engaged in the profession and with your fellow colleagues. It never ceases to amaze me how many of my friends are often dealing with the same professional or personal issues that I am.

Likewise, it is rewarding to give advice to my fellow colleagues on issues that I have previously experienced or resolved. Your networking environment can be through professional associations, your job, church, school, or just your friends. Remember, those contacts could be very valuable in your career. The friends you make through networking can last a lifetime.

Sixth, sustain contact with your mentors and mentor others. Mentors are special, unselfish individuals who provide advice throughout your career. They are advisors, confidants, and trusted nonjudgmental friends. Sustain and savor the relationships with your mentors as your career grows and develops. As your career continues, you should become a mentor to colleagues and friends who will need your wisdom. That will be the payback for all the valuable advice you gained from your mentors.

Your career will be exciting and rewarding. It will be filled with many unknowns, turns, triumphs, and challenges. I never could have predicted all of the accelerated technology inventions and the transformation that have occurred in our profession. And yet, somewhere, I found that following these six principles helped guide me along the way. There will be unknown challenges and new opportunities ahead in your career. If you focus on your success, always place others' interest ahead of yours, strive for excellence, and follow the advice contained in this book, someday you will be writing letters of sage advice to those who follow you. Remember, a successful career is not just a destination, but a journey that is so very rewarding.

Sincerely,
*Harold N. Godwin*

# Stuart T. Haines

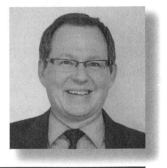

*Seek Support, Contribute to Your Team,*
*and Focus on the Patients' Needs*

Even though he is unlikely to admit it, Stuart is one of the clinical trailblazers in the profession. Working in the pharmacy department of a Veterans Administration hospital during college ignited his passion for progressive clinical practice and led him to the realization that his career path would not be a traditional one. His impressive career has involved innovative clinical practice in diabetes management and other specialty areas. As a board-certified pharmacotherapy and ambulatory care pharmacy specialist, Stuart feels that credentials are important to pharmacists because they provide a competitive edge and establish credibility with fellow members of the health care team. Stuart has achieved fellow status in the American College of Clinical Pharmacy (FCCP), American Society of Health-System Pharmacists (FASHP), and the American Pharmacists Association (FAPhA).

Stuart is Professor qnd Vice Chair for Clinical Services in the Department of Pharmacy Practice and Science at the University of Maryland School of Pharmacy in Baltimore, Maryland, and Clinical Pharmacy Specialist—Primary Care at the West Palm Beach VA Medical Center in West Palm Beach, Florida. He earned his bachelor of science degree in pharmacy from the Massachusetts College of Pharmacy and Allied Health Sciences and his doctor of pharmacy degree from the University of Texas at Austin. He completed a pharmacy practice residency at Brigham and Women's Hospital in Boston and an ambulatory care residency at the University of Texas Health Science Center in San Antonio. His letter advises that *to blaze your trail in clinical practice, focus on the patients' needs, seek support, and contribute to your team.*

Dear Young Pharmacist,

It was great to meet you the other day at the conference. Your questions were very insightful and got me thinking! On the plane ride home I began to reflect on the trials and tribulations I faced in my own practice.

Starting a new clinical service is never easy, and it is not surprising to me that you have run into some roadblocks. While every institution and organization has its unique culture, the circumstances you described are not unusual. Human nature is surprisingly consistent! Most of us resist change. So hang in there. Be persistent. You are on the right track.

You asked about how I started the diabetes management service. To be honest, I cannot take credit for creating the service—it was a *team effort*. That is probably the most important piece of advice I can give you. Don't attempt to go it alone—indeed, you will be doomed if you try! I suppose in the "old" days it was possible to hang a sign up and create a service your own way—but health care delivery is a team sport now. Health care organizations are incredibly complex and, unfortunately, slow to change. Nonetheless, learning how to enlist the support of key people within your organization is critical. Navigating the organizational politics and figuring out who are the key players sometimes can be tricky. To be successful, you will need the support of people not only in your department but throughout the organization.

It sounds like your boss is really pushing you to get something started. Although the pressure to succeed can feel like an extra burden, the good news is that you have her support. Believe me, not everyone has that advantage. There are many people who have the backing of the physicians and nurses, but their direct pharmacy supervisor is skeptical or downright antagonistic. Be sure to use her knowledge of the organization and experience as a leader to help you! Seek her advice and, if you are not doing so already, meet with her regularly. She has a vested interest in your success, but she probably has a lot on her plate. Sometimes young practitioners can feel abandoned because they have all this pressure to get services started but do not get the direction and encouragement they need. Remember that your boss hired you because she believes you have the knowledge and skills to get the job done. She might not check in with you regularly thinking that you can handle everything on your own; so, unless you tell her, she will not be aware of your struggles. Do not be afraid to ask for her help, and don't expect her to make the first move. Communication is a two-way street.

I am not surprised that you are getting some push back from the nursing staff. I have had the good fortune of working alongside some very dedicated nurses and dietitians who welcomed my input. However, some of them feel threatened. In most institutions, the nursing staff is the glue that makes the place run, and their jobs are not easy. So it is important to understand and be empathetic toward their concerns—do not minimize or bypass them! People have a funny way of being territorial and clannish and pharmacists are no less guilty of this.

Rather than telling the staff what you plan to do and what pharmacists have done at other places, ask them what they need and how you can best serve patients. Start by gathering information about their perceived needs and be open to their ideas. In other words, do not go in with a fixed agenda. When the diabetes management service was first being formulated, I thought my primary role would be to adjust and manage diabetes medications. Wrong! I quickly realized that the endocrinologists, nurse practitioners, and nurses that I would be working with already had advanced knowledge and experience managing patients with diabetes. They were all board certified! When it came to diabetes medications, they really did not need my help. Or at least, they did not need my help for routine things. But there was a subset of very complex patients—those taking medications that adversely impact glycemic control or who had difficulty taking 12 or more different medications a day who could benefit from my services. Moreover, none of the physicians or nurses had much experience with smoking cessation—and, as you know, the combination of diabetes and tobacco use is particularly harmful. So, rather than spending my days adjusting insulin doses and making recommendations about what anti-diabetic agent to initiate, I directed my time and effort toward areas where I could really make a difference. I never envisioned that I would become the smoking cessation guru in the practice or the person who made the "cool looking" medication calendars for patients! Of course, as time passed, the endocrinologists and nurse practitioners did, from time to time, ask my opinion about what agents to use in a particularly difficult patient case. When the nurse educators' schedules were full, they began to schedule some patients with me to initiate and titrate insulin therapy. By listening to and addressing their needs, I was accepted as an essential member of the team. And slowly but surely, I had a significant influence on prescribing behaviors and raised awareness about all sorts of medication-related issues that impacted patient care throughout the entire practice. And, just as importantly, they influenced me! So be open, be flexible, and be a team player. You will accomplish far more.

You asked about credentials and how to establish your credibility. I am a firm believer in residency training and board certification, but not for the reasons you might anticipate. Graduating at the top of your class, completing residency training, and having a string of initials after your name does not really matter to most people. Frankly, most of the physicians and nurses you work with will not understand what it all means. And most of your patients will not care. So why bother? You should not be driven by what other people think but rather by a desire to be a highly competent practitioner. Ultimately that is what people will notice—your confidence and skill! So, I strongly encourage you to pursue board certification, but remember the primary reason for working hard to earn and keep those credentials. It is not about the extra letters after your name, but the confidence in knowing you are at the top of your field.

Good luck. It was truly a pleasure meeting you, and I would be honored if you would keep me posted on your progress. I hope to see you at the conference again next year!

*Stuart*

# Mick Hunt

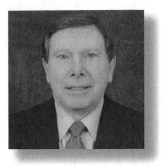

## *Doing the Right Thing*

Impeccable integrity, ethical, thoughtful, caring, and a drive to do the right thing are thoughts that immediately come to mind when those who know Mick are asked about him. He certainly embraces the concepts of doing the right things in his life and his profession. When he is faced with difficult decisions, he approaches them in his naturally thoughtful manner and you can almost see his thinking process including fact-gathering, analysis, and assessing the right thing to do followed by his decision. As he shares here, doing the right thing should become engrained in the fabric of who you are as a leader and a person.

Mick is Associate Professor and Vice Chair of Pharmacy Administration at the Northeast Ohio Medical University College of Pharmacy in Akron, where he led the process to implement a combined master of science degree and administrative residency program. He is formerly Vice President of Pharmacy with Novation, the supply chain management company for the VHA and the University Hospital Consortium. Mick was also Director of Pharmacy at the University of Kentucky Hospital and Lutheran General Hospital in Park Ridge, Illinois.

Mick received his bachelor of science and master of science degrees from the Ohio State University College of Pharmacy and completed a concurrent residency in hospital pharmacy at Grant Hospital in Columbus. He also holds a master of business administration degree from the Lake Forest Graduate School of Management.

Mick offers great advice for the many times that you are confronted with difficult decisions during your career and life: *consider your options carefully and make ethical decisions.*

Dear Young Pharmacist,

I would like to share with you a principle that I have found helpful in guiding my career. It makes common sense and is certainly not a novel idea; but it is one of those things easier said than done. Putting this principle into practice may require a disciplined effort on your part or help from others until it becomes a natural way for you to do things.

"What's the right thing to do?" During my tenure as president of American Society of Health-System Pharmacists (ASHP), that was a question I heard more often than I care to remember from Henri Manasse, the Executive Vice President and CEO of ASHP at that time. Believe me, when you have that question posed to you repeatedly, it changes your way of thinking and the decisions you make. Eventually, however, it becomes engrained into the fabric of who you are as a leader and a person. Although I felt that I had embraced this concept of always trying to do the right thing during my entire career, Dr. Manasse really drove it home to me and raised my awareness to a new level.

Doing the right thing means that you make decisions and do things based on considering a perspective larger than your own. It means considering what is best for another individual, a constituent group you serve, the organization, or the profession—even if it is not in your personal best interest. It means not reacting to a situation in a manner you will later regret, but thinking through what an appropriate response would be.

Many examples of doing the right thing that I experienced as president of ASHP involved making difficult funding decisions when the economy took a downturn. Funding new programs was critical; but so, too, was upgrading computer capabilities, promoting pharmacists as medication management experts, moving to electronic-based publications, promoting medication safety, and retaining an excellent staff. There were many worthy endeavors to pursue, but we had to consider diminished funds. Those were tough decisions, but the ASHP Board of Directors and staff worked together in the best interest of its members.

I recall a time as the director of pharmacy in a 700-bed hospital in suburban Chicago when I began reporting to a new manager. She was the former vice president of nursing and was just promoted to vice president for patient care services, with pharmacy services included in her scope of responsibility. Our relationship at that point was cordial, respectful, and a little distant. At the time, our hospital system was in negotiations with another hospital system in the area—a system of comparable size with a flagship hospital similar in size to ours. Soon after I began reporting to her, I was asked to investigate why their flagship hospital could function with a much smaller pharmacy staff than we had—and that, of course, an explanation was needed immediately. A quick on-site visit to the other flagship hospital predictably revealed that their pharmacy services were at a much lower level than our services. The difference in service levels was documented, analyzed, and reported to the vice president. However, I wanted to take that investigation a step further and compare our department staffing with comparable hospitals offering a similar level of pharmacy services, keeping in mind the short turnaround time requested. So, I turned to data available through the ASHP Resident Match Program, thinking that these hospitals shared a common minimum standard of practice to meet residency accreditation standards. A quick analysis of pharmacy staffing per occupied bed provided a very high-level comparison. Our hospital had a separate corporation for ambulatory services and our outpatient pharmacy operation did not report to me. Believing that other hospitals surveyed had probably included their outpatient pharmacy personnel in their staffing levels, I included our ambulatory care pharmacy staff in our total staff even though they were technically not part of our hospital. When I explained my reason for including our ambulatory staff in my calculation, our vice president was amazed. She asked why I would do that because she would have never been aware of it. I told her that I thought it was the right thing to do, to which she responded, "You just bought instant credibility," and then explained how important that was to her. That move, although I potentially put myself and our department at a disadvantage, changed our whole relationship. I became one of her most trusted managers, and she later wrote a strong letter of recommendation for my next position. It was a risk; but it was the right thing to do.

Always give credit where credit is due and shine a light on the person who steps up to the plate. Toward that end, whenever our pharmacy department achieved a noteworthy goal, I always invited the person primarily responsible for that accomplishment to attend one of my regular meetings with the hospital chief operating officer to give a report. Rather than taking credit for the accomplishment myself, I used this opportunity to recognize the contributor for their achievement on an important stage and to encourage that type of leadership among our staff. I was frequently asked why I would do that because other managers did not follow that practice. Again, I always felt it was just the right thing to do.

If you are considering an action that you think is something you will worry about in the future, it's probably not your best option. As your career progresses, you will often be confronted with dilemmas regarding what you should do in a certain situation—they may be large or small. Will you make a decision or take an action that is always in your best interests even if it means stretching the truth a little? Will you take a short cut to get ahead at someone else's expense? Will you respond to a conflict in a manner that is satisfying to you at the moment, but one that you will regret in the long run?

Although it can be difficult, you will be well served to follow the principle of *Always Try to Do the Right Thing*.

Respectfully,
*Mick Hunt*

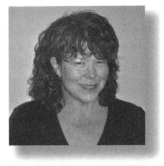

# Kathi S. Lucas

*Follow Your Heart, Seize Opportunities, and Realize There Are Always Trade-Offs*

Kathi is an example of a woman who "has it all." She is a dedicated pharmacist and has still found the time and energy to be very active in Boy Scout leadership (even after her son completed scouting). Kathi has always consciously prioritized her family equally with her career as her letter describes. Before the advent of the concept of transitions of care, Kathi worked collaboratively with nurses, physicians, social workers, and administrators as the bone marrow transplant clinical pharmacist who took care of both the ambulatory and inpatient stays. She is also an example of a clinical practitioner who moved into formal leadership positions but maintained her BCOP certification and indeed did chose to return to clinical practice.

She completed her bachelor of science in pharmacy at Auburn University and her master's degree in public health at San Jose State University. Kathi is currently the outpatient pharmacy regulatory compliance pharmacist at Stanford Hospital and Clinics.

She gives this superb advice: *Follow your heart, seize every opportunity, and know that there will always be trade-offs.*

Dear Young Pharmacist,

It seems that I have come to that time in my life when I am supposed to give out some wisdom instead of gathering it up. I am writing to you because I want to share some things I have learned on my journey as a pharmacist in the hopes that it will make your own journey easier.

My first job in pharmacy was a compromise. Fresh out of pharmacy school and newly married I was faced with a huge change. My new husband's job took us from a city in the southeast and the university teaching hospital where I did my clinical rotations to a small town in California. It was 1975, and the doctor of pharmacy program in California was the hottest thing in the pharmacy world. I expected to take everything I had learned, from satellite pharmacies and rounds with doctors to the computerized IV labels and use it wherever I went in California. Enter reality. Small rural hospitals (even if they were in the mecca) did not necessarily operate like a large university teaching hospital. The nurses wrote down the medications they wanted for patients, and the pharmacy sent up a 5-day supply in the dumbwaiter without ever seeing a diagnosis, a laboratory value, or even the nurse.

I chose to work at a small independent retail pharmacy instead of the local hospital. It was not my dream, but it turned out to be a wonderful first pharmacy job. I could talk to patients, and the only doctor in town was happy to discuss the patient's medication if I felt another choice would be better or if there were interactions. I even took medication calls for the office when the doctor was out of town. I learned a lot about running a business, getting along with an experienced staff of diverse older people, hiring and firing, and working in a community. This experience enabled me to grow and gain valuable career skills.

In 1980, newly divorced, I moved to a city because I felt that I had learned all I could in the small town retail store, and I wanted a bigger challenge. I had the opportunity to go back to a community hospital that had satellite pharmacies with pharmacists who were out on the floors making contact with the physicians. I really wanted to be a satellite pharmacist, but I took the central pharmacy position. It was not perfect. I really wanted to get back into hospitals and was certain that if I did not take this opportunity and waited for the perfect position, I would never get back into clinical practice. Within two weeks of my hire, there was an opening that enabled me to get back to the bedside. I worked with a fantastic group of young clinical practitioners and migrated from the entry pool to a permanent position in the intensive care unit (ICU) pharmacy. I learned that it is important to make the best of opportunities as they offer themselves. This experience impressed on me again the lesson that no job is perfect, and you have to make trade-offs.

My next move was due to layoffs. Even as I was going through the grieving process, I knew that this was an emotional reaction, but it did not keep me from feeling lost—as if I had no identity. A young clinical practitioner encouraged me to apply for an open position and helped me with my resume and interview techniques. My lesson learned here was that when one door closes, another door will open; sitting in the dark is scary, and your friends are hugely important in helping you through the dark.

I never dreamed that I would get back to a teaching hospital. I had already learned from my last experience that if I did not try, it could not happen, and if I did, it very well might. So I applied and was offered the job. I learned that those years of going the extra mile, volunteering for committees, and doing extra projects not only gives personal satisfaction, but also will help prepare you for the next step on your journey.

Going to the university teaching hospital required working the night shift rotation again, working in general medicine not in the ICU, and there was a 20 percent cut in pay. The schedule and pay were a compromise, but getting back to a teaching hospital was the most important thing for me, so I chose to follow my heart.

There was a new program starting right along with me. Bone marrow transplant had two beds and wanted a pharmacist to attend rounds daily. No one else on staff was interested. Here was an awesome opportunity to do something new, something exciting that would call on everything I knew and push me to learn more. These patients were so sick that my ICU skills were a very welcome addition to the team. Learning the oncology portion of the job, which was actually small compared to the medical aspects of managing the patients, was not a problem. I realized how important it is to embrace opportunities as they come along.

I spent 10 wonderful years in bone marrow transplant, but our practice model included providing clinical services 24 hours a day, 7 days a week. My son was 8 years old and showing signs of not doing his homework if left in afternoon daycare. When I was home, evenings with homework were not good, and the evenings when I was not at home were worse. I wanted a fixed day off to volunteer at my son's school. I loved my clinical position, but for my family's sake I needed the stability of a more fixed schedule. I had been offered management opportunities but was never interested because it seemed that I talked to my managers only when there were problems. They tended to be reactive and stayed in their offices. I did not think management was a good fit for me.

The new department managers had management styles that impressed me. They were willing to listen and encourage staff, include the staff in decision making, and guide the staff in making good choices in their day-to-day activities as well as their careers. Even more impressive was that they were out of their offices seeing what I needed. I knew that I could learn from this team and be successful as a manager with their mentoring. It was with a great deal of excitement that I accepted my first management position.

The Operations Manager position was my favorite of all my career positions. Yes, it was crazy; yes, I took work home with me; but at the end of the day I felt good about helping other people do their jobs. I learned how important a great team was to a successful management role, and how much value there is in mentoring (both receiving and giving).

I owe much to my mentors, and to my "best friends" at work. I would like to thank them all for their support and encouragement through the not-so-great times and their celebrations in the wonderful ones. Without them, the journey would not have been anywhere nearly as interesting, or as much fun. I am glad the journey is not quite over yet.

The following is some advice I would like to share:

- Make friends at work, and hold them dearly. Pay attention to them and celebrate their accomplishments. They will help you through the bad times and help you celebrate the good times.

- Nothing is perfect. Decide what is really important to you and be willing to accept compromises on the things that are not as important. You are not entitled to the perfect job—you have to work for it.

- Remember that time flies, and things change. Sometimes something you thought was a show-stopper may morph into the best opportunity you ever had.

- Smile, and enjoy and embrace what you have. If you have a great attitude all the time, you will find that things are actually pretty good even if they are not perfect.

I believe that the journey is the destination. I have found a great deal of joy in my journey as a pharmacist. Yes, a few frustrations from people who did not see the world or value people the same way I did, but it has been a great ride.

Let me leave you with one last thought—an anonymous quote that hangs on my wall— *The hardest part of starting a new journey is taking a leap of faith right at the beginning.*

Thank you for your time and attention to my letter, and best wishes for a wonderful journey of your own.

*Kathi*

# Henri R. Manasse, Jr.

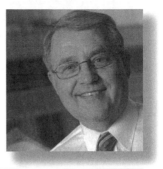

## *Social Relevance, Purpose, and Legitimacy*

Many have experienced life-enriching conversations with Henri, and if you enjoy time with people who make you think, Henri will be at the top of your list. He often brings a social, moral, and global perspective to conversations and has a unique ability to connect those perspectives to practical aspects of your life. He is intensely devoted to his family, profession, friends, and his societal purpose. Here he draws from his personal family history through which he powerfully states that a profession must exist in a bigger social context.

Henri retired as the Executive Vice President and Chief Executive Officer of the American Society of Health-System Pharmacists (ASHP). He has served as Vice President for Health Sciences and Professor at the University of Iowa, Interim Vice Chancellor for Health Services University of Illinois at Chicago Medical Center, and Dean and Professor at the University of Illinois, College of Pharmacy. He continually worked throughout his career to improve patient care by serving in leadership positions for professional organizations including the American Association of Colleges of Pharmacy, the Federation International Pharmaceutique, and the National Patient Safety Foundation.

Henri received his bachelor of science degree from the University of Illinois, his master of arts degree from Loyola University, and his doctor of philosophy degree from the University of Minnesota. In recognition of his contributions, he received the Harvey AK Whitney Lecture Award, ASHP's highest award for health-system pharmacy, and received several honorary doctor of science degrees from major universities. He was inducted into the Institute of Medicine of the National Academy of Sciences in 1996.

Here Henri encourages you to *consider your role as a professional in a free and democratic society.*

Dear Young Pharmacist,

I am a son of the Holocaust. What does THAT mean, you might ask? Simply put, my mother and father were victims, but fortunately, survivors of the terror inflicted on them by the Nazi army when it occupied The Netherlands from 1940 to the end of World War II in May 1945. Both of them were in and survived Nazi concentration camps—my father at Westerbork in the Netherlands and my mother at Ravensbrück in Germany near Berlin. My father's parents were both murdered at Auschwitz; hence, I never had the pleasure and joy of growing up with grandparents on my father's side of the family. Many family members on my father's side also perished at the hands of the Nazis.

You might now ask why I am sharing this deeply personal part of my family's history. Again, simply put, these realities were at the foundation of my psychological, social, and moral development as a child and ultimately extended as I grew into adulthood. They served as the backdrop and context of my socialization as an individual. To this day, the stories from my parents and other family members who survived the almost five-year occupation of my birth homeland, and the experiences that I have had around this family history, have had a major impact on my thinking, acting, and perspectives. I have visited several Nazi concentration camps, have read many books and articles around the Holocaust theme, have been to the United States Holocaust Memorial Museum in Washington, DC, and the Yad Vashem Memorial in Jerusalem, and have talked with other Holocaust survivors. I have visited the many memorials, museums, and the historic sites related to the Holocaust in Berlin, the heart of the Nazi government and military. I have also been to the national cemeteries where the liberating and sacrificial soldiers from the United States and Canada are buried.

My family immigrated to the United States in March 1954, the same year that the United States Supreme Court rendered its decision on *Brown vs The Board of Education of Topeka, Kansas*. My memory of the graphic newspaper images in the *Chicago Tribune* of the race riots that resulted from this decision is still vivid in my mind. My mother actually questioned whether the family had made the right decision to come to America. Later in life when I was a young academic, I learned that Jewish professors who had lost their jobs in German universities during the expansion of national socialism in Germany attempted to be employed by American universities but were not successful due to the strong anti-Semitic sentiments abounding in majority white universities. Many of them were received by predominantly and historically black universities in the Jim Crow South. I also lived through the race riots in Chicago after the assassination of Martin Luther King, Jr. in 1968. In fact, the west side of Chicago where I was finishing my pharmacy education was literally on fire during that time.

These deeply impressive family and experiential roots in my background were not lost in my thinking about pharmacy, pharmacy practice, and pharmacy education during my early professional development and throughout my career. You might then ask, how can that be? Well again, simply put, our pharmacy world (e.g., practice, education, regulation) exists within a bigger social context.

The issues of social justice, equity and equality, social worth and significance, professional power and influence, and social obligation and accountability are all applicable to pharmacy as a profession and to our daily lives as pharmacy professionals. Our profession exists only to the extent that the broader society grants us the social privileges associated with access to medicines, their appropriate distribution, and ensuring their proper use. That privilege is undergirded by fundamental ethical, moral, and legal principles linked to the Hippocratic admonition that we do only good for our patients. Pharmacy's social object must be focused on the application of scientific evidence and clinical judgment and experience related to appropriate medicines management and use in society. To the extent that our profession meets this obligation, we will have social relevance, purpose, and legitimacy.

The Nazi era in Europe and the American experience in slavery and civil rights are specific examples of their respective societies getting morally and ethically off track. These abridgements of a moral and ethical compass resulted in the deaths of millions of people and embedded hatred and strife that continues to have lasting reverberations in our nation and the world. These atrocities were perpetrated while the majority said or did nothing. I am reminded of the words of Edmund Burke, the Irish parliamentarian who stated:

> *"The only thing necessary for the triumph of evil is for good men to do nothing."*

These matters also have implications for our profession. Our professional associations work hard at advocating for continuous advancement, thus identifying those policy issues and professional challenges that demand speaking the truth and creating desired futures. But that advocacy work always has as its backdrop some historical truth. For example, the disastrous compounding problems that occurred at the New England Compounding Center cast a dark pall on our profession.

I want you to think deeply about your role as a professional person in a free and democratic society. I know I have burdened you with some heavy issues, but I have done that purposely. I want you to think about your civic, as well as professional, engagement in society. I also hope that you will give deep thought to issues of social justice and equality and always focus on doing good. To these ends, I wish you a rewarding career and continuous happiness in your chosen profession.

I'd like to end my message to you with my favorite quote from Shakespeare's *Hamlet,* as Polonius admonishes his son:

> *This above all: and to thine own self be true.*
> *And it shall follow as the night does the day.*
> *Thou canst not then be false to any man.*

Blessings and the best of all to you my dear mentee!
*Henri R. Manasse, Jr.*

# RADM
# Thomas J. McGinnis

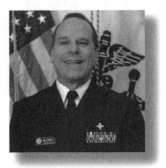

*Build the Strongest Foundation
of Knowledge and Skills That You Can*

How many of us, when presented with three job offers, would choose the lowest paying? Not many, I suspect. But that is exactly what Rear Admiral (RADM) Thomas J. McGinnis did after graduating from pharmacy school, choosing to pass up two more lucrative offers to join the United States Public Health Service (PHS). Tom has spent his entire career in the PHS and, looking back on it, he has never regretted that decision.

Tom's letter describes his remarkable career at the U.S. Food and Drug Administration and later taking the helm of the U.S. Department of Defense's TRICARE Pharmacy Program, which provides pharmacy care to almost 10 million members of the seven uniformed services and their families. His work has provided many interesting challenges and many opportunities to improve our citizens' health. One of his most memorable and rewarding experiences was his deployment to storm-ravaged areas along the Gulf Coast in the aftermath of hurricanes Katrina and Rita.

Tom currently serves as Chief, Pharmaceutical Operations Division, responsible for pharmacy operations of the Defense Health Agency. He earned his bachelor of science degree in pharmacy from Rutgers University and a certificate in general administration from the University of Maryland. He is a graduate of the Federal Executive Institute.

Tom's advice to young pharmacists is to *record your observations, milestones, and lessons learned over time; build the strongest foundation of knowledge, skills, and contacts that you can; and build a strong personal foundation.*

Dear Young Pharmacist,

In a world full of career choices, I commend you for choosing the profession of pharmacy. Pharmacists are involved with all facets of the health care system and knowing what is available and how to achieve meaningful and rewarding goals early in your career will help ensure your success.

While still a student, I began my career with the U.S. Public Health Service (PHS) in the Commissioned Officer Student Training & Extern Program at the St. Elizabeth's Hospital in Washington, DC. This three-month internship program gave me my first insights into the PHS and what pharmacists were capable of doing. After graduating from Rutgers, I had three job offers: one from the pharmaceutical industry, one from a chain pharmacy, and the PHS. I chose the lowest paying job with the PHS and have never regretted that decision. Little did I know, nor even imagine at the time, that I would spend the next 36 years performing a variety of different, interesting, and challenging PHS assignments.

From very early in my career, I remember volunteering for projects and working closely with the PHS Chief Pharmacy Officers, RADM Dick Church and RADM Richard Bertin. At the American Society of Health-System Pharmacists (ASHP) Midyear and the American Pharmacists Association (APhA) annual meeting, I would help with the PHS exhibits and recruiting activities. An extra pair of hands was always needed to work on important pharmacy projects, and I learned a great deal from performing this volunteer work. I was introduced to other pharmacists at these professional meetings, and I developed a network of pharmacists and allied health professionals that was extremely valuable as I advanced to higher levels throughout my career. These Rear Admirals were very positive thinkers and always expressed things in a positive way. Everything was possible, and their enthusiasm was an inspiration to junior officers who met them. I counsel you to seek out positive people and learn their ways. While they exude enthusiasm, these leaders also seem to have ice in their veins and do not fear making mistakes. They know how and when to adjust their goals quickly and would assume whatever role was necessary to accomplish the goal. They do not care about the glory and make sure those working with them get the recognition. In my own experience, I was always amazed at how they would take the time to listen to any young officers who wanted to meet with them and offer them career-enhancing advice. They embraced the idea of being a role model in the PHS and always acted with the utmost integrity. They seemed to know that their legacy as a Rear Admiral in the PHS was not so much what they were able to accomplish, but that they were helpful to others. I still enjoy having breakfast periodically with many of these retired admirals who will listen to my problems and offer me words of wisdom.

My career with the PHS allowed me to move around within an agency and still have the ability to grow and work in different specialty areas. PHS officers are a part of Department of Health and Human Services (HHS) and have a mission to protect, promote, and advance the nation's health and safety. Of the many career opportunities in the PHS, one of the most challenging but most memorable experiences occurred after hurricanes Katrina and Rita hit the Gulf Coast in 2005. I was deployed to central Louisiana to direct a PHS field medical station that provided medical services to 250 patients that were relocated because of the hurricanes; we took care of patients under very austere conditions until the state's infrastructure was re-established.

My focus today is the pharmacy benefit management for all uniformed services. The PHS is one of the seven uniformed services. Eight years ago, I was asked to work with the Department of Defense and run the newly formed Pharmaceutical Operations Directorate in the TRICARE Management Activity. The TRICARE Pharmacy program is robust and includes many program areas, but ultimately this program provides a pharmacy benefit to all eligible active duty service members and their families, National Guard and Reserve members and their families, and retirees and their family members and covers 9.6 million individuals.

I want to leave you with three challenges. First, think about what you would like to be doing 10 to 20 years from now and write that down in a notebook. It does not have to be long, eloquent, or complex, and the only requirement is that it must be genuine. Continue to record your thoughts, observations, milestones, and lessons you have learned over time. Then, about every 4 to 6 months return to your notes and read what you wrote and reflect on your goals. Record the events or personal milestones that you have reached or still need to reach to help you grow professionally or even the things that may cause you to question your goals. It is very helpful to share your thoughts and feelings with friends or mentors. You should refine your goals as opportunities come along. The cycle of writing, reflecting, discussing, and successively refining your goals will help you to chart your professional growth and keep you on course.

Second, build the strongest foundation of knowledge and skills that you possibly can. Do not underestimate your abilities, and do not be intimidated by the different socioeconomic backgrounds or ranks of others. I have found many great generals and admirals to be humble in dealing with those of lessor military rank or rank in society. You will need to take personal initiative to seek mentors and professional contacts to build your personal knowledge base and network. Do not let any opportunity pass you by. New technology and tools, such as Linked In, further multiplies availability to create this important network and to keep current. You must appreciate and understand each person's personal and cultural point of view because unless you can effectively communicate with each patient, peer, or the public, your training and personal development will not serve you very well. Do not underestimate the value of common sense to learn how to apply your vast amount of knowledge to fit any given situation.

Finally, build the strongest personal foundation that you can. Always remember that your family and friends are the most important things in your life, no exceptions. You will also need to develop a routine and stick to it to keep both your body and mind strong. Learn very quickly that it is not just about you—it is about you, your patients, and your community and how these three interact. I believe that every successful career should begin by finding a way to serve those who are underserved and most need the talents you possess. Helping those special needs patients in Louisiana was the most rewarding thing I did in my 36 years of service, and it made a lasting impression. I challenge you to find a way to give something back as you develop your career.

A strong foundation of knowledge and skills, when tempered and guided by your heart, will most certainly keep you true to your goals. I am confident that whether you follow a similar road to mine or whether you simply serve one patient at a time to the very best of your ability, you will have a very rewarding career.

*Tom*

# Paul G. Pierpaoli

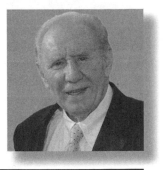

## *Do Not Ask More of Your Staff Than You Are Willing to Give*

In talking with Paul you might be struck by his communication style. His Harvey AK Whitney address, *An Iconoclastic Perspective on Progress in Pharmacy Practice,* is evidence of his straight-forward style. Paul is a consummate leader who is willing to fight for what is in the best interests of not only his staff, but his patients. He is willing to challenge the status quo no matter what the personal cost. He continues to be a dedicated mentor to numerous students, residents, and young practitioners, sharing his philosophy and experiences. Paul has given unselfishly of his time to an array of professional organizations and has also served as ASHP President.

Prior to retiring, Paul was Senior Vice President, Pharmacy Practice, McKesson Medication Management. He had previously served as Director of Pharmacy at Rush-Presbyterian-Saint Luke's Medical Center, Medical College of Virginia Hospitals, and the University of Connecticut Health Center.

He received his bachelor of science in pharmacy from the University of Rhode Island and completed a residency and master's degree at the University of Michigan. Prior to retiring, Paul was Senior Vice President, Pharmacy Practice, at McKesson Medication Management.

He indicates in his letter: *Do not agonize over work/personal life conflicts, as trying to compartmentalize your professional life and personal life can be a futile experience for a truly dedicated professional.*

Dear Young Pharmacist,

Perhaps you are a pharmacy resident, a student, or a recently graduated practitioner. Regardless of your status, you have one common and immutable calling that binds you to your peers. Specifically, it is a mandate to provide the necessary leadership to improve and expand pharmacy practice. It is an obligation—not a recommendation.

Having walked the same path as you over 55 years ago, I am delighted to share some of the highlights of my own journey, as seen through the prism of leadership development. I came to hospital pharmacy after a chance encounter with a pharmacy school friend. He had recently resigned from a part-time student position at a large hospital pharmacy department and recommended that I apply. I got the position and never looked back! For me, the hospital setting provided a unique learning environment where I could regularly apply and reinforce the theory of pharmacy practice and pharmacotherapeutics gleaned in the classroom and laboratory. I was able to "connect" instantaneously. It was exciting and gave me an immense sense of pride in my chosen profession.

At the beginning of my senior year, a professor recognized my passion for hospital practice and suggested formal post-graduate education and training. Hospital pharmacy residency training was then in its early stages. My professor, a University of Michigan alumnus and analytical chemist, strongly recommended Michigan, with its well-established master's degree program and structured residency training program in the University of Michigan Hospital's pharmacy department, directed by Dr. Donald Francke, a national and international leader in hospital pharmacy. He was also a founding member of the American Society of Health-System Pharmacists (ASHP) and the editor of the *American Journal of Hospital Pharmacy*. I took his advice and completed a two-year residency and master's degree.

Dr. Francke was the consummate mentor and preceptor. Despite his responsibilities as a director of pharmacy and his active involvement in ASHP and the international pharmacy community, he always managed to find time for his residents, both on an individual and collective level.

His mentoring was rooted in critical thinking. He constantly reminded us of our roles as future leaders and admonished us to challenge the status quo of hospital pharmacy practice. Perhaps one of the most salient aspects of our mentoring was acquiring a conceptual approach to problem solving rather than a "quick fix" or one-of-a-kind solution. The importance of understanding the context of a problem was always a part of our problem-solving efforts.

For me, residency was a defining social and professional life experience. It set the compass for what turned out to be a fulfilling and satisfying career in hospital pharmacy. I realized that the essence of such training and experience involves developing a strong sense of who you are and what constitutes your strengths and weaknesses. Take on the mantle of practice leadership, make a personal commitment to changing pharmacy practice, and develop a personal professional philosophy.

As a resident, I became acutely aware of the consequences of the absence of leadership in many other hospital pharmacy departments. It was then that I made a deliberate choice to make my contribution to the profession as a director of pharmacy and mentor. After much hard work and determination, I took my first position as a director at age 26, less than two years after having completed the residency.

I subsequently took on a succession of directorships in three community hospitals over a course of less than 6 years. My personal philosophy, as a manager and leader, for better or worse, was not to ask more of my staff than I was willing to give. Needless to say, such a philosophy led to enormous stress and dysfunction in other aspects of my life. I realize now the heavy toll it took on my wife and family. The dislocation of my family and my separation from them every time I changed positions was very stressful. I had not anticipated the enormous amount of time and physical and mental stress involved in taking on the position of director. In the absence of corporate relocation expenses or reimbursement, each change resulted in a higher level of family debt. Our family quickly learned to look at each move as an opportunity to start a new beginning.

This chapter in my life also helped to point my career toward directorship positions in academic health science centers, especially those with schools of pharmacy. I found that my tenure in community hospitals did not fill a deep-seated need to be in a milieu that also stressed education, research, and innovation in health care. My experience of 34 years as director of pharmacy in three academic health centers has provided a great sense of accomplishment and satisfaction. Even more rewarding, however, has been the opportunity to teach and mentor hundreds of pharmacy students and residents.

Touching the lives of new practitioners and helping to shape the profession's future through these relationships has provided an unparalleled bounty for me. My colleagues and I shared a vision for a new and changed future for pharmacy and the patients we serve, which far surpassed any material accomplishments or recognition. It came at a price, however, especially in the form of the time and effort that it usually entailed. For the dedicated mentor, many an evening's dinner or family outing has been forgone in the course of taking an opportunity to mentor a resident or student. It is a habit of the heart.

Each time I changed career positions I found a new set of significant, and sometimes daunting, challenges. In fact, my entire career has been a composite learning and growth experience generously peppered with disappointments and adversity.

I want to leave you with the following general observations:

- Take every opportunity to embrace change or to be in an organization or an environment that is changing. It can get you out of your comfort zone and foster self-discovery and self-knowledge, which can strengthen you against adversity, disappointments, and setbacks. Eleanor Roosevelt said, "*we gain strength, and courage, and confidence by each experience in which we really stop to look fear in the face.*"

- Seize every opportunity to become a mentor. The satisfaction is incomparable as you progress in your career. It guarantees your legacy to others.

- Do not agonize over work/personal life conflicts. Trying to compartmentalize your professional obligations and personal life can be a futile experience for a truly dedicated professional.

- Stand up and advocate for pharmacy. It is a noble profession. Take every opportunity to make changing pharmacy practice an obligation.

Remember, we all are leaders. Best wishes for your ongoing journey in leadership.

Sincerely,
*Paul G. Pierpaoli*

# Pamela A. Ploetz

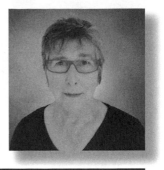

## You Can Only Control Your Choices

If you know Pam, you know that she cares about you. Pam is a lifelong learner who sees the whole picture and has a unique ability to put it in perspective for you. She is a great coach and mentor focusing not only on successful careers but also on success in life. Pam summarizes a few life lessons in this letter. She draws from her personal experiences, shares her thoughts on the situations life can sometimes hand you, and reminds you that you are only in control of your decisions.

Pam spent most of her career at the University of Wisconsin Hospitals and Clinics in various roles, progressing from staff pharmacist to Associate Director of Pharmacy Practice, Education, and Research, and Director of Pharmacy Practice Residency. She was also Clinical Associate Professor for the University of Wisconsin School of Pharmacy. She served her profession as President of the Wisconsin Society of Hospitals and the Pharmacy Society of Wisconsin. Additionally she was Chairperson of the Wisconsin State Pharmacy Examining Board. She received her bachelor of science degree from the University of Wisconsin School of Pharmacy.

Pam teaches you to *take time when making core decisions and make sure they are the ones that are important to you.*

Dear Young Pharmacist,

We have all heard, "If I only knew then what I know now." Obviously we can't go back, but we can learn from those who have been there. Life is a series of choices. From a very early age we are all forced to make them. How do we avoid making bad

**103**

choices, and how do we make the good choices that move us further along in our careers?

You are not in control of most things presented in life. Life hands you situations, and they are yours to handle. You do not control which issues you will face, but you can control your choices of how to handle them. Some of the decisions you will make will have little or nothing to do with what is really important. Others really do matter, and you have to think them through carefully.

When I was young, my mother was diagnosed with multiple sclerosis. She had a very difficult life and died when I was in college. This experience shaped my life from the get-go. I learned very early on that nothing assures you of good health. Many would say that they know that, but it forced me to explore and identify what was important *to* and *for* me. My dad encouraged me—I would say forced me—to do many things outside my comfort zone such as going to camp (and weeping with homesickness), playing softball with no natural athletic ability, taking swim lessons in the morning when I hated cold water, and staring at pea soup for hours sure that I would hate it. You get the picture! These and many more experiences plus thinking about what I liked or did not like resulted in greater self-knowledge. Some were negative, and some were positive. Upon reflection and looking for patterns, I discovered that my miserable feelings at camp were experienced once again when I applied to colleges far away from home. This then became one of my core decisions—I wanted to remain close to my family. Did that close doors and limit opportunities? Perhaps, but when those core decisions are made, then new opportunities and experiences present themselves. Decisions and choices become easier when they fit self-knowledge.

Self-knowledge also led to a career change. Early on, my practice was in the clinical areas, and I loved helping patients with their medications and working with the medical staff. I was a bit of a control freak and thought that there were definite improvements that could be made in the practice setting, the schedules, you name it. I was young and, believe me, I had answers. So I took on administrative roles only to learn that I was soon doing a less-than-optimal job taking care of the patients and showing little patience with the people I was hoping to lead into greater clinical practice. I eventually realized that I could make a clinical difference in an administrative position. But I also learned two important lessons:

- Do a few things well and make sure that they are the ones that are important to you.

- When leading others, help maximize their ability to know core strengths and talents to achieve their goals and to lead in whatever role they choose.

It is not how you get there that is important but that you get there.

So my advice to you is to experience all that you can as soon as you can. Do, do, do, and do some more. Travel to the other side of town and to the other side of the world, read all you can and not just professional journals, talk to strangers, listen to music and not just what you like or think you like, try a new restaurant, go to the opera, try a new sport, participate in a flash mob, etc.

To go and do should be the mantra. But then going and doing cannot be the end—you must pause and ponder. Take time to put the puzzle together. Figure out what is important to you. What gives you the most peace and pleasure? Keep testing and keep growing. Evolution is the key. From this knowledge, one can make better decisions and by owning those choices you can change them. When they feel good, they become core values. Do not be mistaken; this is not an easy process. This took me an eternity of thinking and pondering, framing the positive and negative impacts of events in my life, exploration, and connecting the dots of various experiences to arrive at my core decisions. This is a solitary journey because this is all about you, and you should not take this process lightly. People are so busy doing that taking the time to ponder and wonder about life issues is often lost. One needs to pause and make time to reflect. This is so essential and critical in the journey to knowing yourself and reaching those few core decisions that are important to you and to your life. I might add that knowing yourself thoroughly and knowing you did your best, offers a chance at peace later in life.

I had a second insight when I retired, which, by the way, is a huge life transition. There were five other women at a similar place in their career, and we decided to become a support group for each other. Thus, we became T.I.T.—Tootsies in Transition. We gathered monthly to share experiences and find out what each was doing to survive the transition. One day the conversation revolved around happiness: Were we happy? The group's elder statesperson said she knew the answer—decrease expectations. What? Where do goals and objectives and return on investment, for example, fit? She smiled and went off to another meeting. In retrospect, this observation would have totally improved my life. But there is no time like the present. So now when I am down or feel off, I check my expectations. The small exercise of checking your expectations can change many situations if not to happiness, then certainly to make them tolerable.

Some final thoughts for you are:

- Take the time and effort to thoroughly understand yourself and what is most important to you.
- Do what matters and keep the big picture perspective.
- Don't re-live all your decisions.
- Do the best you can at the time, learn from the experience, and go forward.
- Not happy? Check your expectations.
- Listen, listen, and listen.

My best wishes to you on this wonderful life journey.

Sincerely,
*Pam Ploetz*

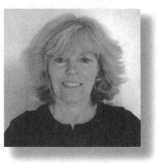

# Barbara Schlienz Prosser

---

## *Networking Is Not Overrated, It Is Underestimated*

If you were to ask members of Barb's team about working with her, you would hear terms such as fairness, caring, supportive, doing the right thing, and networked. Barb is a leader that understands the value of a team, getting things done as a team, and the importance of a network. As you will read, she learned these lessons early in her career and has used them in many aspects of her life.

Barb most recently served as Vice President of Clinical Operations for Critical Care Systems/Accredo and has more than 25 years in the home infusion industry. She has helped develop and shape this industry through volunteer leadership positions in organizations such as the National Home Infusion Association, the American Society of Health-System Pharmacists, and the Joint Commission including serving as a Surveyor in the Home Care, Ambulatory, and Network Accreditation programs for the Joint Commission. She received her bachelor of science in pharmacy from the University of Florida, College of Pharmacy in Gainesville.

Barb's letter focuses on the value of networking. Through her personal experiences, you will relate to situations where you will benefit from your professional or personal network for help or support. As Barb states, *it's never too early in your career to network.*

---

Dear Young Pharmacist,

"What's the best advice I can offer?" That is an interesting and difficult question! As I reflect on my career in search of a response, I believe many things shape my best advice: organizations, people, family needs, mentors, and even lost opportunities. But the people and the connections stand out by far.

The people I have met along the way have opened endless doors for me. Walking through those doors has led me to new job opportunities including opportunities to lead for change. I have had the privilege to work with the best in our profession, make changes in policy, and redirect energy and focus during committee work. These people had the greatest influence on my career. Thus, the focus of my advice is to meet and network with the leaders in our profession. Those connections will provide you with the ability to move beyond your safety zone and explore new avenues.

Networking is not overrated; it is underestimated. My first job in the home infusion industry ended badly. I was with the company two years and had worked my way into a management role. The company was sold, and the new management and I did not see eye-to-eye. I was ultimately let go and found myself jobless and coincidently expecting my first child. I took some time to reassess my situation and work through all the emotions you might imagine related to loss of a job. It was a time of transition in my life; I was nervous about being jobless, and nervous about how being "let go" would influence my ability to find a satisfying job. The natural inclination would be to find a job in my comfort zone, but I knew I needed more. I was about to be a first-time mom and wanted some time with my child. I wanted flexibility and not to be tied to a weekend schedule. I was married to a nuclear pharmacist who worked weekend nights and slept during the day. I clearly needed to reinvent my job description.

I thought long and hard about where I wanted to go in life and in my career. I believed I had found my niche in home infusion and wanted to stay in the field. I also needed to factor in my soon-to-be family and how I would need to balance that. I realized that the traditional hospital rotating schedule was not optimal for me, nor did I want a full-time commitment. I basically wanted a part-time, meaningful career to keep me engaged in my profession as well as home with my family. So I reached out to my network to see what was out there. I spoke to colleagues in academia, long-term care, and in retail. Then, I reached out to a consultant I had worked with during my last days at the company. He seemed to have the flexibility and challenge in his job that I was looking for. The company brought him in to retool our processes and workflows, and I had spent considerable time with him on the job learning and listening. (Today I still joke with him, claiming that his report was the reason for my demise. We remain close friends and still open doors for one another.) I picked his brain about opportunities and reinventing my career and asked if he had contacts that would be beneficial to me. This conversation led me to a part-time position as an accreditation surveyor. My networking was successful. I became part of a group of new surveyors that helped to define and shape what is today the premier standard-setting organization for the home infusion industry. For 10 years, I worked part-time while spending time with my two young daughters at home, and yet learning every day. During my years surveying, I met many leaders in the industry and made valuable connections. I gained experience and knowledge by seeing a new organization and new ways of doing things in each survey I conducted. I still serve as a committee member for the accreditation organization and forging new connections.

Do not wait until you need a network to develop one. Start now. There are many ways to do this. Membership in professional organizations was the second most important step I took in moving my career forward and making it meaningful. Professional organizations are the mecca of networking. Many of the same people I met while surveying were also leaders in our professional organizations. Through their encouragement and opening a few more doors, I became involved in the American Society of Health-System Pharmacists and the National Home Infusion Association. Their energy, commitment, and forward thinking showed me that I could make a difference and how to channel my passion to make change. One of the connections I made through networking at meetings brought me to my computer today to write this letter. A connection with a man who was a mentor, an inspiration, a friend, and a provider of hugs at times! Working on committees, writing papers, taking on my own leadership positions have allowed me to help shape and be part of changes in our pharmacy world. I have had the privilege to chair and work on committees that helped to shape the home infusion industry legislation initiatives, define accreditation standards, and establish practice guidelines for our practitioners.

Maintaining my membership and activities in the professional organizations while working part-time enabled me to stay connected. As my children grew older and entered school, I took a job at a national home infusion company as the Director of Clinical Services. I entered this job just as the company was expanding. As a result, I found myself at the start of something big. I had to build a department to take this company to the next step. I relied on my network and was able to build what I thought was the dream team of clinical operations. Without those past ties, I would have relied on recruiting web sites and whatever resumes happen to find their way to me.

My daughters are now grown and pursuing their own careers. One daughter is a wildlife biologist and the other is a public health major in college. My advice to them has been the same. Network, ask questions, explore all opportunities, design your own career path, and then find the people who can help build it.

As my older daughter received her college diploma and I listened to the Dean conferring the degrees on the students, I was struck by part of the verbiage used, "With all the rights, privileges, and honors thereunto appertaining."

Our designation as registered pharmacists comes with a set of rights, privileges, and honors. They are ours for the taking, but we have to find them and define them. Make change, challenge established ideas and processes, and help move your profession forward. I was not the stellar student in pharmacy school nor did I win awards such as "Most Likely to Succeed." But I have had the most rewarding career I could have imagined, and I totally attribute it to the people I met along the way.

Don't let your profession happen to you; you be the one to make things happen!

*Barbara Prosser*

# Max D. Ray

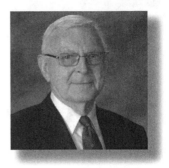

## *Grow, Create, Lead*

Max continues to be adroit in not only thinking about critical issues facing pharmacy but in putting his conclusions into publications so others can benefit. This skill is evidenced in his 1997 Harvey AK Whitney Lecture, *Letters from the Edge*, in which he writes three imaginary letters on what is meant by professional practice, the qualifications, and activities required. The letters are from 1940, 1997, and 2040. He has seized various opportunities throughout his career to contribute, moving from practice leadership and college faculty, to professional organizational staff, and culminating in being a college of pharmacy dean.

His bachelor of science degree in pharmacy is from the University of South Carolina and his doctor of pharmacy and master's in hospital pharmacy degrees are from the University of Tennessee. He completed a two-year residency at Methodist Hospital in Memphis. Max currently serves in a contractual capacity as a consultant to the American Council for Pharmacy Education and is part time faculty at the University of Tennessee College of Pharmacy.

In his letter he states that *serving a purpose bigger than ourselves is more important than embellishing your resume.*

Dear Young Pharmacist,

You will receive this message interleaved with several others, all written by experienced pharmacists whose only motive is to help you achieve your potential as a leader in pharmacy. Through our respective careers, we have all come to understand that leadership is required of us—it is not an option. If our hard-learned lessons can assist you in becoming an effective leader, our goal will be achieved.

Here, then, are my thoughts on the topic of leadership.

Leadership requires a purpose. It is not sufficient to say "I want to be a leader," or "I am preparing myself to be a leader." What completes that thought? For instance, you want to be a leader in improving health-system pharmacy. That would clearly state the general direction in which you might lead. Remember that the phrase *to be a leader* is an incomplete thought—it requires a predicate (in other words, action)!

Leadership should serve a larger purpose. To what purpose are you, as a pharmacist, willing to devote yourself? Can you say clearly that you are motivated by some deeply held sense of professional responsibility? Is it more important to pursue that responsibility than it is to embellish your resume? Do you care who gets credit for accomplishing a goal? *Servant leadership* is a term Robert Greenleaf uses to describe this altruistic form of leadership (*Servant Leadership: A Journey into the Nature of Legitimate Power and Greatness*).

Pharmacists have a moral responsibility to provide leadership on behalf of their patients. Dr. Doug Hepler reminded us that this is part of our covenant with society ("Pharmacy as a Clinical Profession" in *Am J Health Syst Pharm*). It really is not acceptable to opt out of being a leader when we are actively engaged in providing patient care. To speak up and to take forceful action (e.g., when we become aware of potential medication problems) may require moral courage. But to *not* provide leadership in such instances is an act of moral cowardice and professional malfeasance.

Leadership also requires creativity. Effective leaders always have alternate pathways to achieve their goal. To envision those alternate pathways requires creativity. Some of us are more creative than others, but I believe creativity (much like leadership) can be nurtured and cultivated. By trusting our creative abilities, we will be more effective leaders. To broaden your thinking about creativity and the creative process, I recommend Mihaly Csikszentmihalyi's *Creativity: Flow and the Psychology of Discovery and Invention* and Daniel Boorstein's *The Creators: A History of Heroes of the Imagination.*

Great leaders are dragon-slayers. While in fiction some leaders may have faced actual dragons, in more mundane settings (for example, in a health-system pharmacy setting or a patient-care setting), this translates to confronting problems *as individuals* and struggling with those problems until we find a solution. There is no substitute, in my view, for the *personal quest* experience—pharmacists who have the courage and stamina to wrestle problems to the ground, even at great personal inconvenience. These pharmacists are the ones who will become strong leaders.

Leaders create change. Rather than being controlled by, or victimized by, change, an effective leader actually creates change. Leading an organization (or a group of individuals) through a process of change presents great challenges. The body of literature on change management is voluminous and rather daunting, but I recommend (as a place to start) John Kotter's *Leading Change*. His eight stage process of leading change has been tried and found useful by many leaders in a variety of organizations.

Leadership is an ad hoc process. During the course of a day, most pharmacists find themselves switching from a position of *followership* to *leadership*, depending on the circumstances. It is important to realize this and to accept it. In the clinical setting, we often follow the lead taken by a physician or a nurse, but then step up to take a leadership position when medication-related decisions are being made or discussed.

Leadership entails practicality. It is much more than a state of mind or a theoretical way of thinking. It requires action. To make our maximum contribution to society as health-system pharmacists, we will need to invent new ways of going about our practice—both as individuals and as pharmacy service departments. We need leaders who understand the down-in-the-trenches realities of pharmacy practice and have a sustaining vision for how to make our greatest contributions. We need leaders who can shift quickly and establish and maintain equilibrium between the *big picture* view and the *on-the-ground* view that characterizes our most effective leaders.

As leaders in pharmacy, we must always be aware that we sometimes get it wrong. Frequently, our mistakes have more to do with timing and in overestimating the level of support we have built for the desired direction, rather than with the direction itself. To persist in the face of evidence that one is on the wrong course is a common pitfall. To avoid this, we should continually seek advice from those we trust, apply continuous quality improvement principles, and then temper our judgment based on our best evidence. Let me share with you a personal example of one such wrong-headed direction I attempted to take.

When I was the pharmacy residency program director at a major medical center, I became convinced that one year of residency training was inadequate to produce the level of maturity required for practice in most clinical settings. I developed a plan for a new residency training model, entailing 18 months of general clinical experiences and 6 months of specialty experience. (The standard American Society of Health-System Pharmacists [ASHP] designation of postgraduate year [PGY1 and PGY2] programs had not yet been established.) After presenting this plan to our staff (including those who served as preceptors in our residency program), I thought I had sufficient support to proceed. We launched this new model and were successful in filling our quota that first year. But it soon became obvious that I had seriously misjudged the preceptors' support. I had not listened carefully enough to their concerns. (We ultimately aligned our program with the new ASHP-established PGY1–PGY2 model.) Was my vision wrong? Perhaps not. But I was wrong in overestimating the level of support.

Finally, leaders must be capable of self-renewal. John Gardner's *Self-Renewal: The Individual and the Innovative Society* states that perhaps the leader's greatest challenge is to create "a system or framework within which continuous innovation, renewal and rebirth can occur." Young leaders should think about their own process of self-renewal. This process requires reaching deep within oneself, drawing on the self-assurance that comes from slaying dragons, getting in touch with one's creative process, and continually reflecting on when to lead and when to follow.

As you think about your professional career, the goals you want to achieve, and the contributions you want to make, I encourage you to consider carefully where you want to work. Look for environments where leadership potential is valued and nurtured, where creativity is encouraged, and where the collective vision of your co-workers is one that you can enthusiastically support. Find that sort of environment and then grow, create, and lead.

With all best wishes,
*Max Ray*

# Jennifer L. Riggins

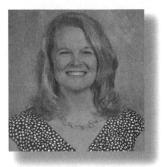

*There Is No Growth in a Comfort Zone
and No Comfort in a Growth Zone*

Jennifer is a busy industry professional, association volunteer, avid sports fan, and mother of three young sons. She was initially drawn to the profession of pharmacy because it paid well, offered many diverse career options, and provided the flexibility that she valued. She freely admits the factors that first attracted her to pharmacy are different from those that keep her excited about her work now. She has spent her career in the pharmaceutical industry, working in various roles in medical information and medical affairs. While she is passionate about her work now, her first role as a neuroscience medical information specialist proved to be anything but her dream job. Her letter provides insight into dealing with such a scenario and other challenges that may come your way. She advises you to be courageous and bold, and to look for growth opportunities even if they take you outside your comfort zone.

Jennifer is currently Advisor, Global Medical Channels and eCapabilities in Customer Engagement and Medical Affairs at Eli Lilly and Company in Indianapolis. She has been with Lilly since 1993, serving in a number of progressively responsible positions in medical information, medical communications, and global medical customer solutions. Jennifer received her doctor of pharmacy degree with honors from Butler University. Jennifer provides sage advice: *stay true to yourself and find the right balance in your professional and personal life.*

Dear Young Pharmacist,

I often think back to the time when I chose to become a pharmacist. Why did I make that choice? What impact did that choice have on my life and would I make the same choice again? I can unequivocally say YES! I made the right decision. I went into the field of pharmacy because it seemed like a good, flexible job for a woman. Pharmacy jobs paid well and offered a lot of different options. I stayed because I enjoyed my colleagues; I loved my varied roles and responsibilities, my work environment, and the flexibility of my schedule. Here is my story and my advice to you as a young pharmacist.

More than 20 years ago, I joined the pharmaceutical industry in the medical information department supporting a new antidepressant. I hated it! I hated the neuroscience (NS) area but loved medical information. A colleague joined the area at the same time and focused on anti-infectives. He really enjoyed the NS area and not the anti-infective area, so we switched responsibilities. I became the "antibiotic Queen" providing information to health care providers (HCPs) so that they could make more informed patient decisions. I loved it! Eventually, I moved into other medical affairs' roles focused on scientific communications and business operations such as strategy, people, process, and tools/technology. However, throughout my various technical and supervisory roles, I stayed closely connected to medical information and HCP customer-facing roles—my passion-focus areas.

Here are my top 10 pieces of advice—learned on the job (some the hard way!).

First, love what you do—you spend too many hours at work not to. Follow your passion—not the money or the title. Those will come on their own. One of the best things about my responsibilities has been the global nature of my roles. I thoroughly enjoy collaborating, supervising, and learning from colleagues around the world. As a result, my viewpoints, experiences, and values are richer and more meaningful. A colleague once said to me, "Isn't it cool that we can walk through our company's halls and hear multiple languages, see multiple ethnicities, and experience such diversity of thought and experience?" Indeed, it is!

Second, supervisors make a difference! I worked with some good, GREAT, and not-so-good bosses. I learned something from each one. From one not-so good boss, I learned to make certain that I focus on others' needs and not on myself and to listen and be open to a different opinion. From the great ones, I learned how to be my best self. Stick with the great ones. Try to find the "golden nugget" and learn what you can—even if it's what NOT to do.

Third, be bold and courageous. Take a chance on growth experiences that will be meaningful to you. I took some chances along the way. Sometimes they panned out; sometimes they did not, but I am glad that I took them. I have a plaque on my desk that says, "There's no growth in a comfort zone and no comfort in a growth zone." I have grown a lot, and it has been uncomfortable at times. Make sure you grow and are open to possibilities.

Fourth, get involved, collaborate, and form partnerships. External collaboration has been so important to my career and my personal satisfaction. Early on, I became involved with external not-for-profit professional organizations and schools of pharmacy. I started by precepting, mentoring, and developing PharmD students on their drug information rotations. Soon, a colleague and I partnered with a university to start a Drug Information Specialty Residency. Talk about a big job! We poured a lot of love, sweat, and tears into the program. We became accredited and at the time, we were only the second program with an industry component to achieve American Society of Health-System Pharmacists (ASHP) accreditation. I volunteered for a professional organization, served as a speaker, committee chair, workshop chair, etc., and was eventually elected to the DIA Board of Directors. Through those experiences, I built my professional network, gained external insight and perspective, brainstormed ideas, showcased strengths, and developed additional skills such as collaboration, negotiation, and influence. Best of all, I learned from newly developing leaders (students and residents) as well as already seasoned professionals.

Fifth, seek advice from trusted colleagues. During a time of discontent with my job and thoughts of changing positions, I met with trusted colleagues and mentors to help me think through the personal and professional impact of potential decisions. As a result of one particular mentor's profound words, I stayed with the company but was better prepared for the battles ahead. Her advice to stay the course and think long-term versus in the moment had a powerful impact on my career and family. Words are powerful; use them wisely!

Sixth, stay true to yourself. I work for a fairly conservative company. When I began working there, the unwritten dress code was blue, black, or gray suits and white shirts for men and dark suits or dresses for women. I like a lot of bold color so I wore bold-colored suits. Sometimes people would stare and I would just smile. Thankfully, times have changed. My organization is now much more accepting of diverse styles, thoughts, and actions and encourages employees to bring their whole selves to work, not just the part that fits the mold. Be authentic, but self-aware. Honor your commitments and know your limits. Keep a life-work balance that fits your needs. Keeping this balance is one of the ways that I stay true to myself. My co-workers know that when I have to choose between family and work, family comes first. Have confidence in yourself and what you stand for—it will give you the courage to make a difference.

Seventh, be a change agent. We sometimes have to drag co-workers kicking and screaming into "the new." Be an early adopter of changes such as technology, process, etc. In my first industry role, I was an early adopter of a new global process for creating medical letters. Being an early adopter allowed me to be a leader in shaping my work environment and deliverables and, ultimately, afforded the opportunity to shape the medical information industry by globalizing our medical information business. My current role brings technology into the business and enables the business to better connect with HCPs. Change can cause disruption, but the individuals who adapt most quickly tend to be the most successful. They become a resource, function at higher levels more quickly, and can better envision how technology, processes, and business need to evolve.

Eighth, own up to your mistakes and failures. Take responsibility and accountability for your mistakes. When I was choosing to make a career move, I decided to communicate this confidential information to two of my direct reports. My supervisor did not agree with that decision. "Proper" communication was very important to her. I knew that, and it hurt our relationship for a year. I learned a lot from that misstep. We all make mistakes, and all have failures such as missed deadlines, failed projects, or an incorrect prescription. Correct what you can. Apologize if you need to. Learn from what did not work. Move on. When you are solving problems or dealing with specific issues, come prepared with solutions. This will demonstrate critical thinking skills, creativity, and proactive problem solving. You will be seen as part of the solution and not just part of the problem.

Ninth, have humility in the face of success and adversity. I am a firm believer in the power of humility to bring people together. An attitude of service and a willing spirit go a long way. A successful person does not need to flaunt successes and knows how to say, "I was wrong." As pharmacists, we are typically very successful, driven people. We must be careful to show confidence, not arrogance, and realize that our circumstances can quickly change. True humility is refreshing and energizing, especially for one's teammates and collaborators.

Finally, ask for forgiveness, not permission. If you know it is the right thing to do, the risk is minimal, and the value is substantial, then, just do it. If you are successful, then it is a win-win situation. If you are not, then ask for forgiveness and own your mistake. Be empowered, and you can make a difference.

Good luck on your journey,
*Jen*

# Michael D. Sanborn

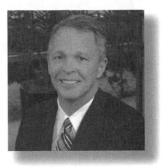

## *Making Difficult Career Decisions*

Mike is the leader that every board of directors wants in a senior executive role in their organization. He is the ultimate professional and a great leader with a tremendous ability to develop and execute a strategic vision. Mike's successful career is a testament to these abilities. His other admired characteristics include his thoughtful and reflective analysis of difficult situations. Thus, the thoughtful approach to making difficult decisions that he shares in his letter is not a surprise to anyone that knows him.

Mike currently serves as the President and CEO for Baylor Medical Center in Carrollton, Texas. His previous experience includes direct patient care and administrative and pharmacy leadership positions in large health systems and academic medical centers. He certainly gives back through his involvement in a number of community and professional activities including serving in leadership roles for the Metrocrest Chamber of Commerce, American Society of Health-System Pharmacists, American Heart Association, United Way, and others.

He received his bachelor of science and master of science degrees from the University of Kansas where he also completed his residency training in pharmacy administration. He has enjoyed a very successful career and, of course, has faced several crossroads during his career. From those experiences he offers very thoughtful advice: *objectively analyze the situation and distill the decision down to the elements that are most important to you.*

Dear Young Pharmacist,

Congratulations on choosing a profession that will provide you with an endless number of career opportunities. Some of the most rewarding yet challenging crossroads that you will face will be related to job opportunities that come your way in part because you are a pharmacist. For that reason, I would like to share three stories of my more challenging career situations and then provide three important pieces of advice for you to consider when you are faced with a new job opportunity.

My first story is about how I got into management in the first place. It was completely happenstance and initially against my will. My first job out of pharmacy school allowed me to fulfill my dream of being a clinical pharmacist in cardiology at a large academic medical center. I literally could not wait to go to work every day to be involved in the direct care of patients. About six months after I started this job, the lead cardiology pharmacist left and I was asked to lead the team (which essentially meant that I was responsible for developing the schedule and resolving issues). Despite some reluctance, I enjoyed it more than I thought I would. Six months later, my supervisor, who was responsible for managing all 27 clinical pharmacists on the various patient care teams, took a job at another hospital. Despite my being only one year out of school, I was approached by the assistant director of pharmacy and asked if I would interview for the clinical supervisor position. The decision to do so was challenging because I knew that I might be leaving a position that I truly loved for something with which I had very little experience. Nevertheless, I interviewed, was offered the position, and chose a path of management. That decision transformed my career.

My two-year residency in pharmacy administration leads me to my second story. After residency, I stayed on as an assistant director, but my ultimate goal was to become a director of pharmacy. After a few years, I was offered a director's position in Florida that I accepted and sincerely enjoyed. Several years later, an opportunity arose with a large company that provided health-system pharmacy management services nationwide. This was a very unique but unorthodox opportunity for me to manage pharmacists and technicians in pharmacies all over the country. To this day, I consider that role to be the most challenging and rewarding job that I have ever had. In every instance, my team was charged with going into very distressed pharmacy operations and turning them around very quickly. The administrators in the facilities that hired us were genuinely grateful to see the positive transformation of pharmacy practice in their hospitals. I would probably still be in the same job today if it were not for one critical event that occurred after a long week of travel. At the time, our division of the company had experienced tremendous growth to include pharmacies in 40 states, Puerto Rico, and Canada. To cover all of these hospitals, it was common for me to leave home very early on a Monday morning and get back on Friday or Saturday. Despite this often grueling travel schedule, I was enthralled with my job. One Friday I arrived home and as usual greeted my wife and two sons. My three-year-old was excited to see me but looked up at me and said, "Daddy, where do you live?" Those five words were a tough blow to my heart and precisely the moment that I knew a career change was required.

My final story focuses on what some might say is the reason I "left" pharmacy. My relationship with my current employer has provided me with many opportunities and promotions. I started out as the director of pharmacy for their university teaching hospital and over time moved into my current role of chief executive officer (CEO) for a 235-bed community hospital. My decision to accept a leadership position that was entirely outside of pharmacy did not come easily. Throughout my career, I have observed a significant contrast between the profession of nursing, which tends to permeate virtually every aspect of health care practice, versus pharmacy, which generally tends to be singularly focused on pharmacy practice alone. In fact, a large number of pharmacy directors across the country report directly to nurses, which often struck me as odd. Frankly, it is rare for us as pharmacists to step outside of our pharmacy comfort zone into a role that is minimally rooted in what we studied in pharmacy school. Admittedly, there is comfort and job security associated with this wonderful profession for which we have trained and have years of practice experience. When I was asked to consider leaving this comfort zone to pursue a broader role in hospital leadership, I discussed the myriad of advantages and disadvantages with my wife and mentors. In retrospect, my role as CEO is more rewarding than I ever anticipated, much like my other tough career choices. As a CEO, my ability to singularly influence the actions of physicians, nurses, and, yes, pharmacists has grown exponentially and has ultimately had a positive and measurable influence on patient care at our facility. As a pharmacist, I do not believe there is a greater reward.

There are three pieces of advice that I have learned over the years that can truly help make a very difficult career change decision a little easier. First, make a list of pros and cons associated with staying in your current role and compare them to those associated with the new position. Be sure to include both the professional and the personal benefits. Although this exercise may sound trite, there is no better tool to objectively analyze the situation and distill the decision down to the elements that are most important to you.

Second, always do your best to make sure that you have a good boss. Research shows that the majority of people leave their job because of a poor relationship with their direct supervisor. Do not let this happen to you. During the interview and negotiation process, make sure you have a good understanding of your prospective supervisor's expectations and that you feel your personalities are compatible. Most importantly, try to determine if they have your best interests and success in mind. If you suspect that there is a problem in this area, it might be wise to pass on the opportunity. Always remember that a great boss will end up being a mentor and your best professional advocate.

Finally, keep an open mind about new and different opportunities. These types of career moves often provide the greatest occasions for exponential learning and new experiences. When you think outside the box and take on a role that is somewhat unorthodox, it can be very exciting and rewarding.

In closing, I wish you the absolute best in your career and trust that you will make decisions that will advance not only yourself, but your family, the profession of pharmacy, and patient care.

Sincerely,
*Michael Sanborn*

# Bruce E. Scott

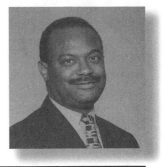

## *If You Don't Have a Mentor, Get One*

Those who know Bruce will attest to the fact that success has not changed him one bit. He is still the same warm, personable, down-to-earth, and humble person he was when he began his career. An accomplished hospital pharmacy director, business leader, and visionary, Bruce exemplifies all the qualities we expect to see in a successful leader. He rose to the ranks of corporate vice president, chief operating officer, and president, and led the practice of more than 3,500 pharmacists, nurses, dietitians, and other health professionals. Bruce was one of the youngest pharmacists elected ASHP president.

Looking back on Bruce's storied career in pharmacy, it is difficult to imagine that anyone would have been qualified to serve as his mentor. Yet, despite his stature in the health care community and his many impressive achievements, Bruce acknowledges the important role mentors played in providing guidance and support on his path to success. Mentors helped him understand the importance of learning, encouraged him to develop a vision for his career, and helped him set and achieve his goals for his term as ASHP president. His positive influence as a mentor to scores of pharmacists will continue to reverberate through the profession for years to come.

Bruce currently serves as President of The CADENT Group, LLC, providing consultative services to health care businesses and provider-related organizations. He has served in executive roles at Allina Hospitals and Clinics, McKesson Medication Management, and Medco Health Solutions. He earned his bachelor of science degree in pharmacy from the University of Wisconsin School of Pharmacy and a master of science degree in pharmacy administration from the University of Kansas, where he also completed a pharmacy residency program.

His advice to young pharmacists on selecting a mentor is clear: *Mentors are invaluable as a sounding board, providing an objective point-of-view and direction in support of your success.*

Dear Young Pharmacist,

Looking back on my career, it is obvious to me that I owe much of my success to mentors. Yes, mentors! My advice to you is, if you do not have a mentor, get one.

My first mentor was the high school band director at the large, inner-city public school I attended. Despite being raised by a great mom and teacher, and having many teachers in my family, I did not know how to be successful in school. Although I understood that grades were important and I achieved good grades, my mentor helped me understand the difference between good grades and learning. I enjoyed hanging out with friends and while I knew I had to take responsibility and be accountable for my decisions, he highlighted the power of suggestion and the danger of "group think" among friends. This mentor helped me prepare for life post high school and helped me to recognize that there were many landmines along the way. Success was preparation for a future without stepping on the landmines.

I was enjoying my first job as a pharmacist when my next mentor, a pharmacy leader at the University of Wisconsin Hospital, asked me about my vision for my career. At that time, I was delighted to be finished with school and working in a job that paid more money than I had ever made. My vision extended as far as my next shift at work. Pam had experience on the journey ahead of me and had observed many pharmacists along the way. She urged me to consider a different career path and, through our many conversations, I became committed to a career that I probably would have never pursued: A career in pharmacy leadership. She not only helped me create a vision for my future, but also helped me develop and execute a plan that included graduate school and a residency. I did not seek this mentor, but I am forever grateful that she chose to mentor me.

Mentors have also helped me think through and accomplish goals. I was fortunate to serve as the President of the American Society of Health-System Pharmacists (ASHP) from 1999 to 2000. Soon after I was elected to this position I received a wonderful letter from Dave, a long-time mentor and past president of ASHP. He congratulated me and urged me to think about strategies to accomplish my goals during this period when I had the chance make a difference. We discussed the importance of my communication as president, building support for goals, and being mindful that I had a responsibility to work with the board and staff to accomplish goals during the three years that I would serve as a presidential officer, not just the year as president. He helped me focus my thoughts on what I believed to be important, what I could realistically achieve during my term, and the strategies to achieve them.

My mentors have shared my successes, disappointments, and listened to my ideas, which have ranged from great ideas to not-so-great ideas. These conversations often start with a call from me saying: "You will not believe this!" or "This is what I am thinking." Our discussions generally include handling difficult situations, feedback on an issue, career changes, skills I need to acquire, and general life plans. The key is that there is no topic that is off limits. Sometimes the most valuable lessons learned were a result of discussing situations that did not go as I planned. Mentors do not make decisions for you. They ask you questions; help you understand decisions, situations, and actions from various points-of-view; and help you envision what is ahead for you on your chosen path.

There are many factors to consider in choosing a mentor, but I think your personal comfort with the person and the ability to have open and honest conversations are most important. You need to share your most vulnerable thoughts and situations, and the mentor has to provide honest feedback. In the beginning, you should communicate frequently. Over time you will find the pattern, style, and time for communicating that works for the two of you, such as my standing breakfast at national meetings with Sara, another of my mentors. Do not hesitate to ask someone to work with you as your mentor because you think that they are too busy or you are afraid to bother them. Often, you will find that people are honored and delighted at the opportunity to help you. The opportunity to give back is important to most people.

Mentors have been, and continue to be, very important in my life. I sincerely believe that you will find great value in having mentors. This is especially true in today's environment where many of us are accountable to annual goals and scorecards, and fewer organizations are investing in training and development programs. Mentors are invaluable as a sounding board, providing an objective point-of-view and direction in support of your success.

Best of luck,
*Bruce Scott*

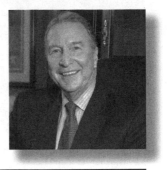

# Ronald H. Small

---

## *Find Your Passion and Pursue It with a Sense of Urgency*

In getting to know Ron, you will find him very principled and willing to be candid about his opinions. Ron epitomizes being his own person. He is one of the first people to justify and achieve being a Chief Pharmacy Officer and thus positioned himself at the senior administrative table. Since retiring, he has become a Certified Executive Coach (CEC) to pursue his passion for leadership development by creating and utilizing centers of knowledge and excellence in health care processes.

He serves as a primary faculty for the Pharmacy Leadership Academy Leading for System Reliability in Safety and Quality Module as well as co-faculty for the leadersINNOVATION Masters Series Strategy and Tactics: Creating Transformational Change course. Although for most of his career he did not venture far from his North Carolina roots, now that he is retired he is traveling the world in his new role. Ron is currently a consultant with Joint Commission International and Joint Commission Resources.

Ron's bachelor of science in pharmacy and master of science in business administration degrees are from the University of North Carolina. He advises that *an achiever has to assume the burdens and rewards as well as be bold and courageous.*

---

Dear Young Pharmacist,

I was born and raised in rural North Carolina. The values instilled by my parents throughout my upbringing were the best "advice" I have ever received. I learned from them to be reluctant to use the "I" word, so in sharing some of my life experiences I am very mindful that my stories are not necessarily a recommendation to follow my model.

My Momma was the most important person in the world to me and the primary source of my values, beliefs, and my life's passion. I say "was" because her life was taken in a health care facility at the hands of well-meaning health care workers, including physicians, nurses, pharmacists, respiratory therapists, and others. Mistakes caused her preventable death. That tragedy provided some important learning experiences for the facility, for me, and for those health care workers who cared for her. So, even in her death, Momma was still teaching valuable lessons.

Let me share some learning experiences that helped shape me and I trust will be of some value to you. Recognize that this advice is based entirely on my own meandering experiences.

When I was about 15 or 16 years old, Momma asked me what I wanted to do with my life. To fully understand my response, you should know that no one in our family had ever been to college. I told Momma that I would go into the Navy because I thought the uniforms were cool. She said, "Is that what you really want to do?" I told her, "No, not really. I want to help people." I really wanted to be a doctor, which many of you in pharmacy can relate to. She suggested that I find my passion and pursue it with great urgency. The family could not support my dream financially, but she believed in me. She suggested that I look in the mirror and believe in myself.

While bagging groceries at the local food store, I had the good fortune to meet Homer Andrews, a community pharmacist, who asked if I was interested in changing jobs. He needed a person to make deliveries and do other odd jobs for his drugstore. At the time, I did not comprehend the role his mentoring would play in my life. I certainly never forgot his professionalism, his truly caring spirit for others, and his accepted responsibility to be a good community citizen. When I expressed my gratitude for his mentoring, he said that we should always serve and mentor each other. After that experience, it became obvious to me that I had to find a way to go to pharmacy school at the University of North Carolina (UNC) so I, too, could help people and fulfill my passion.

Having confidence to achieve a goal can also come from underestimating the goal's challenges and barriers. I assumed that all I had to do was apply to school. I really was naïve. Well, I made a positive mistake. This sounds like an illogical statement, but it was true. I told everyone that I was going to Carolina to pharmacy school before I applied. You can image my surprise when I learned the process for getting into pharmacy school, and then the shock when I realized the cost. But, I had Mr. Andrews' mentoring, Momma's expectations, and my passion.

I was focused and committed to completing my goal of graduating from UNC. I got a job in the UNC cafeteria, working the breakfast shift. *Every* morning I had pancakes and milk, which filled my stomach for the day. I sold my meal tickets—my pay for working—to fund some expenses. I excelled that first year, and I applied for and received an academic scholarship for the remaining years. I worked and borrowed funds and paid everything back over 10 years following graduation. The moral of the story is to find your passion and pursue it with a sense of urgency by developing focus and commitment to achieve your goals.

My family was very proud of me, and I became the center of attention because I was the only one to go to college. Momma told me, "Be generous in all things, but mostly in sharing joy. Go into this sometimes unpleasant and mean-spirited world with a roaring sense of elation. Be clean in mind and spirit. Bring honor to yourself and family in all that you do. Give to those less fortunate." Momma reminded me to take what I did seriously, but not to take myself so seriously. She insisted that I be true to myself. I give you this same advice.

Having shared my North Carolina roots, I must confess that in my childhood I believe that Andy Griffith was a truly great person. He taught many valuable lessons through his weekly television show, which I never missed. Of course, as I expanded my view of the world outside of North Carolina, I found others who influenced me. Stephen Covey, author of *The Seven Habits of Highly Effective People*, was one of those who taught me a great deal.

In response to the question, *What are the most important tenets for a young pharmacist to be successful in our chosen profession?*, my advice is to find your passion and pursue it with great urgency. Passion can be turned into profound results for us and our organizations and the people we serve if we are focused and committed.

Let me offer the following additional advice. Serve and mentor each other. The power of having those things that we are passionate about affirmed and understood by our colleagues is immense.

Serve society. The uncompromising commitment to recognize that society is our most important focus will remain the hallmark of truly visionary pharmacy leaders.

Be bold and courageous. I remember my first year as a Director of Pharmacy. I wanted to implement a Centralized IV Additive Program and do so within a newly created IV pharmacy. The President and CEO, presiding over what was considered the infamous Capital Equipment Committee, informed me that he was not in favor of spending any money to develop a Centralized IV Additive Program. My request was denied. The following year I returned with the *same* proposal. My request was once again denied. With passion, focus, commitment, and confidence, I returned in year three with the *same* proposal, but this time changed the proposal's title to Single-Dose Injectables. Now, you may think this approach might be something other than bold and courageous. But I had passion, focus, and commitment. The proposal was approved.

Assume both the *burdens* and the *rewards* of the achiever. You cannot shirk your responsibilities. Our profession and the people we serve depend on each and every one of us. The rewards depend on the individual's perspective; from my perspective, I thoroughly enjoyed my career at a great institution. I believe as an organization, and specifically as a department of pharmacy, we made a difference in the lives of the people we served. I, therefore, humbly consider myself an *achiever*.

My personal mission statement, borrowing from Stephen Covey, is, "Live life to its fullest, to learn, to love, and to leave a legacy by making a difference in the lives of the people you touch." I have reaped the rewards, and I am obligated by my beliefs and values to assume the burdens.

I emphasized the word *burdens*—they actually give me pleasure as part of my mission statement. I feel, having reaped the rewards of leadership, that I must share my learning experiences freely. As an Executive Coach, it is my responsibility (burden) to assist the so-called "Big L" Leaders with transformational leadership development for organizational change, for which I again reap the rewards. These rewards enable me to freely coach the so-called "Small L" Leaders. So, from my perspective, the *burdens* are really also rewards because I am doing not only what I should do, but what I really enjoy doing.

Remember not to compare yourself to others and shrink at the reflection. You are unique. What you do will determine how and where you will carry yourself in the future. You should stand tall with confidence and humility of spirit. Do not be timid. Seize opportunity, responsibility, and challenge with zest.

Never, my young friend, turn away a challenge to make yourself and the world a little bit better. That is your destiny. I am honored to share these thoughts with you. Oh, by the way, call your Momma; you will miss her when she is gone.

Sincerely,
*Ron*

# Robert J. Weber

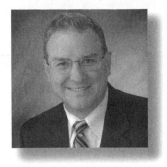

## *My Cancer Experience Taught Me to Put Patients First*

Because of his close call with cancer, Bob is very focused on living in the moment, being a better family person, and putting patients first. He shares a patient's perspective on enduring chemotherapy. He is also very dedicated and passionate about continuing The Ohio State Pharmacy Leadership Training Legacy and is the Director of the Latiolais Leadership Program in the College of Pharmacy. For several years, he has authored and coordinated the monthly Director's Forum column in *Hospital Pharmacy,* which is designed to guide pharmacy leaders in establishing patient-centered services in hospitals and health systems. Bob brings several decades of leadership experience in two academic medical centers both in the service side and the colleges of pharmacy having begun practice as a critical care clinical pharmacist who maintains his board certification.

Bob received his bachelor of science, master of science, and doctor of pharmacy degrees from The Ohio State University, College of Pharmacy. He completed a residency at Grant Hospital. Bob is currently Administrator of Pharmacy at The Ohio State University Wexner Medical Center, Assistant Dean for Medical Center Affairs, Vice Chair, and Clinical Associate Professor in the College of Pharmacy.

Bob gives this great advice: *Please do not let hardships in your life change your course; establish the right course, and you will find out that hardships will be easier.*

Dear Young Pharmacist,

*"Lead your way, keep on strong,*
*moving every day—going further on"*

—Lyrics from *Further On*, Bronze Radio Return, 2013

I hope this letter finds you leading your way, keeping strong, and every day moving further on. This song recently has been buzzing around in my head as I celebrated my 5-year anniversary of my treatment for colon cancer. I feel very lucky to be writing to you now, as I was told that I would only have a 35% chance of being here to do that.

During my chemotherapy, which involved infusions of nauseating medications over two-day periods, I listened to music to distract me. At that time (2008) the Iraq war was in full swing, and two songs served to inspire me: "If You're Going through Hell" and "Mansions of the Lord." I somehow lived vicariously through the soldiers in Iraq; I often saw my battle in the chemotherapy chair similar to our military's door-to-door search missions. My battle was, in some ways, as serious as theirs and when the neuropathy of chemotherapy became so bad that I couldn't function, I was inspired by the fact they were "going through hell" like I was.

But I vowed (and, yes, I really did) to focus on three things if I survived my cancer: being a better family person, putting patients first, and living in the present moment while moving "further on."

Please don't let hardships in your life change your course; establish the right course, and you will find out that hardships will be easier. I hope that makes sense! After a brief discussion about experiences, I will finish with a story that I hope will make a difference for you.

I always thought of myself as a loyal and devoted person—especially when it came to my family. My parents were a very stable couple—my dad a World War II veteran, engineer and my mom a nurse. My wife, Barbara, is a strong person from another stable, hard-working farming family from central Ohio. The examples we had as spouses and parents were from a time that was not so complicated; technology did not influence us, kids seemed to grow up at a normal pace, and careers were more of a 9-to-5 approach. As a parent, I learned very quickly that the definition of a devoted family man has changed. And as my brother says, "Bringing home a paycheck is the entry fee for parenting!" To be a devoted family person in today's world requires you to understand pop culture (something which our parents ignored and dismissed) and to use your emotional intelligence to help your kids with their problems. In talking to my daughter about a problem, I realized that my thinking, analysis, and advice was much deeper and involved than anything my parents had done for me.

You need to be available—emotionally and physically—for your family. This means you need to organize your time in your career to actually attend the class play at 7:30 PM, track meets at 3:00 PM, awards ceremonies at 9:30 AM, and "after prom" at 4:00 AM. Being available means you need to sacrifice your personal time for your hobbies, golf, reading, and even consulting for extra money. You cannot show resentment for this sacrifice because your children will realize instantly that you don't want to be there.

I provide an orientation to our pharmacy students, and always tell them, "At the end of everything you do, there is a patient." My cancer experience taught me to put patients first. I thought I had always put patients first, but in reflecting on my past leadership decisions, I realized I had not. Find out what your patients need and then use that to put them first. Set the expectation with your colleagues by asking "How does this impact our patients?" or telling them to "Put yourself in the patient's place" will help you to course-correct this thinking. Every day, I ask myself how I can help our patients today.

Recently my medical center had to reduce staff, forcing us to change our pharmacist coverage. Following the maxim of putting our patients first convinced us to move a pharmacist from a less acute area to our intensive care units, and risk some political fall-out from a well-known obstetrician who was losing his department's pharmacist.

Before I got sick, I always thought that living in the present moment was a New Age thing as typified by the author Eckhart Tolle (*Awakening in the Now*), who was very popular at the time of my treatments. But I quickly learned that all we really have is the present moment—today, now, while you are reading this. Take a minute now to notice your body. Does your neck hurt from working on the computer? Are you thinking about putting patients first? Are you angry with someone? Your present moment at work should focus on your job;

your times at home should focus on being a better family person. You need to balance this thinking with moving forward, which is hard to do! So think about the present, but then think about how this present can impact what you do tomorrow or the next day.

What does it mean to be in the present moment in your work? For example, I was preparing to go on vacation and was anxiously completing information on my to-do list when an employee (Jim) came to my office. He appeared concerned, and I guess I must have appeared distracted or distant because after we exchanged a few words there was an awkwardness as he left my office. A little voice in me said "Stop! Get to the present moment and away from the vacation. Go find Jim and see what he needs! Something is wrong!" I found him in the pharmacy. He was having difficulty with a physician (who I worked with closely) who was not willing to change an obviously dangerous medication order. When he came to me for help, I was not in the present moment to manage his issue. Now, able to focus on Jim's problem, I called the physician colleague, and we changed the medication order to a safe alternative. Jim was so grateful that I came back to him that he mentioned it 10 years later at his retirement party from the hospital. I felt a sense of pride that I could get back to the present moment and help someone. Always stay in the present—you never know what opportunities you are missing if you do not keep in this moment—now and always.

Focusing on these areas will help you strengthen your personal and professional relationships. It will help you to deal with life's struggles, as you will have forged meaningful and deep relationships with people who can support your most complex emotional needs. The result will make you a better pharmacist, available to help your colleagues and your patients.

Hopefully some of the things I have said will help you find your way, keep on strong, and every day, moving on.

I will finish up with a story that emphasizes the points of this letter. I was very sick early on in my chemotherapy and, frankly, very discouraged. I went to bed on a Wednesday night in June with sense of dread, panic, and despair. On a Thursday morning at around 3:00 AM, I woke up feeling physically strong, with a confident sense of peace and well-being. My wife immediately noticed my demeanor the next morning, and specifically commented that I was a "changed man." This was even more amazing to her because she had seen me the previous night and expressed concern I was not recovering from my chemo treatments. I felt so good that I decided to go pick up my daughter, Natalie, from church camp.

On our way home, she said, "Wow, Dad, you seem a lot better. What is going on?"

I said, "I don't know, Natalie, but I do feel much better."

She then said, "I'm really glad because I had all the kids pray for you!" to which I responded, "Oh, when was that?"

She joked, "You know how the last night of church camp goes! We stayed up all night and talked and watched movies, you know. About 3:00 in the morning. Why do you ask?"

"No reason," I said, feeling a bit shocked and speechless. Then my wife and I looked at each other and smiled.

God bless you,
*Robert J. Weber*

# Sara J. White

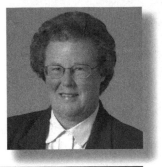

## *Planning for the Future*

Everyone needs a "Sara" in their life! In a very nonjudgmental manner, Sara wants only the best for you. She takes time to understand you and your vision for your career and life, and helps you along the journey to your vision. Her title may be mentor, coach, or friend, but she is always there to support you during the difficult times along the journey and to congratulate you during the good times. In her letter, Sara discusses a portion of life's journey that everyone should plan for—retirement.

Sara currently serves as a faculty member of the American Society of Health-System Pharmacists (ASHP) Foundation's Leadership Academy and a member of the Board of Directors of Omnicell, Inc. Formerly, she served as the Director of Pharmacy at Stanford Hospital and Clinics.

Sara received her bachelor of science degree from Oregon State University and her master of science degree from The Ohio State University, where she also completed her residency. She has served the profession of pharmacy in many leadership positions including President of ASHP. She has been honored as a recipient of many awards including the ASHP Distinguished Leadership Award and the Harvey AK Whitney Award, ASHP's highest award for health-system pharmacy.

Here Sara tells us: *there is no "right way" for a career to evolve, and it is never too early to start planning for the future.*

Dear Young Pharmacist,

Y ou are a unique and special person. There is not another pharmacist alive today with your specific characteristics and potential, and I am happy to share with you my almost 50 years of pharmacy experience. Of course, there are many things I could share with you, but I choose to focus on one you probably have given only fleeting thought—your retirement. It is common to worry about it later; however, if you are like me, you will all too quickly turn around and find yourself at this phase of your life/career. I speak from my experience of being retired almost 10 years but still remaining very active in pharmacy. I want to focus on what you need to do now and what you should track as your career evolves.

No matter what your age, you need to think seriously about the financial aspects of your retirement. Do not be naive and think you can deal with it later. If you retire at 65 to 70 years old, you probably will live at least two to three decades more, and I doubt that you will be able to live on only your Social Security benefits (if it is still solvent). The key to having the money to do what you would like to in retirement, such as foreign travel, hobbies, visiting grandchildren, etc., is to start now maximizing your employer's retirement plan by contributing the maximum allowable including any voluntary plans or open up IRA accounts. Your contributions will reduce your annual taxable income, and the compounding interest over your 30- to 40-year career will add up to significant money. When evaluating a new position, review the benefit plan with regard to the employer's retirement contribution in addition to what you can contribute. After a career spanning several decades, you will benefit from that additional money.

The challenge of retirement is consciously sorting out how to spend your time. When you are working, you long for the freedom that retirement is perceived to bring. As your career evolves, be sure you stay active physically so you keep from slowly gaining weight, which we all know is easier said than done. You need to follow healthy life habits to try to avoid poor health that will restrict what you can do in retirement. During your working career, it is normal to put some of your interests on the "back burner" because there are not enough hours in the day for hobbies or traveling, etc. The key is to document these back-burner things so you do not forget them. As your career progresses, make a note about what you are passionate about or really enjoy as these may be where you want to devote your retirement time. Likewise, knowing what to avoid or minimize is also helpful.

Because I was in a leadership position in an academic medical center, a member of a school of pharmacy faculty, and actively involved in professional organizations including being President of the American Society of Health-System Pharmacists (ASHP), I did not have much free time to think about back-burner activities. My back-burner items were foreign travel, pleasure reading, enjoying the arts (movies, classical music, opera, museums, etc.), playing golf, and hiking. As I reviewed my career, I concluded that my pleasure/passion came from working with young people through teaching and precepting residents. My retirement has consisted of two foreign trips a year, learning about and enjoying classical music/opera and paintings. I really enjoy teaching in the ASHP Foundation's Pharmacy Leadership Academy and have published articles in the *American Journal of Health-System Pharmacy* (*AJHP*) on success skills based on the aspects I taught to almost 100 residents. I co-edited with two young leaders the ASHP *Pharmacy Leadership Field Guide* and completed a four-month ASHP Scholar-in-Residence program that produced a leadership status survey published in *AJHP*, which was redone seven years later and *AJHP* published again. To stay active in the profession but on my terms, I needed to create my opportunities. So, even in retirement you are going to need to take initiative and be proactive.

I began my career when very few women attended pharmacy school. There were some minor discrimination issues. A prime example occurred in my MS/Residency when an assistant director put his arm around me and said he was happy I was interested in clinical because there was no place for women in management. A very interesting comment as my whole career has been in leadership positions. Times have changed, and I found as a leader and a woman that I brought complementary skills to my male counterparts. Another advantage I found were opportunities to be involved in professional organizations because they wanted more women in policy-making positions.

There is not one right way for a career/life to evolve, but the key, I feel, is making conscious decisions that feel right for you and changing them if they no longer work. Because I mentioned I did not have much free time for myself, you might be wondering if I had my career to do over would I make the same choices. *The answer is yes.* I truly enjoyed being very involved in the various aspects of health-system pharmacy. Although it was not by design, I remained single and had no children so I never felt like I was cheating others by my choices. Over a career one faces character-building experiences and difficult moments such as losing the ASHP presidency election for the second time (I stepped back and became the Chair of the House of Delegates before running successfully for the third time for the ASHP presidency), successfully firing employees and withstanding the appeals, surviving several weeks of Drug Enforcement Administration audits, and having to pass the California Pharmacy Exam 25 years after graduation as reciprocation was not available. Through such life experiences you learn who you really are and realize you can achieve anything you set your mind to doing.

Who knows what I will do with my next 10 years of retirement? *The choices are mine.* Begin immediately to save some money and keep track of your back-burner items/passions. Then, when you choose to retire, you can take advantage of the freedom to do what brings you pleasure.

Sincerely yours,
*Sara J. White*

# Billy W. Woodward

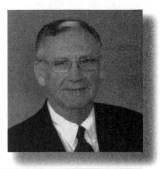

## *Nurture an Enduring Passion for Patients and the Profession*

During any discussion with Billy about his profession, you will almost certainly hear him say that it is about the people we serve and our genuine love, respect, and concern for them; that you must have a "fire in the belly" to fulfill your professional dreams; and that an enduring passion for the patients and the profession will sustain you in your career. His passion for his work and his profession is about a vision far greater than himself: It is about purpose and a better and safer care of patients.

He is currently President of Renaissance Innovative Pharmacy Services, Ltd., in Temple, Texas, and is also a Clinical Associate Professor at the University of Texas. For 25 years he was Corporate Director of Pharmacy for the Scott & White Health System in Temple, Texas, and also served as Director of Pharmacy and Central Services at Methodist Hospital in Lubbock, Texas.

Billy actively supports the pharmacy profession through his work in professional organizations. He has served in leadership positions in the Texas Society of Health-System Pharmacists, the American Society of Health-System Pharmacists (ASHP), the ASHP Foundation, and the International Pharmaceutical Federation. He has received numerous awards including the ASHP Distinguished Leadership Award and the Harvey AK Whitney Lecture Award—ASHP's highest award for health-system pharmacy. Billy received his bachelor of science degree from the University of Texas at Austin.

Billy provides a great insight: *Passion and purpose will provide direction for you during those difficult and challenging times in your career.*

Dear Young Pharmacist,

As you are entering the profession to pursue your personal practice and leadership experience, it is my sincere wish that you achieve your greatest ambitions and dreams for your patients and our profession of pharmacy. I want to share what I learned over four decades as the most critical attribute to ensure such a result. This conclusion became clear to me a few years ago at an American Society of Health-System Pharmacists (ASHP) reception for pharmacy residents when a resident asked the question, "What single factor or trait in your long leadership career do you consider most responsible for your professional success?" This was a surprisingly simple, but penetrating, question that first took me aback. But after a momentary reflection, my answer came quickly, "An enduring passion for the patient and the profession!" For me, this translates to the nurturing of a sincere and passionate belief that a competent, caring, and committed pharmacy team can always make a better and safer tomorrow for our patients!

Through many inevitable ups and downs that passionate vision for our pharmacy team and our patients has never failed to sustain me through difficult and challenging times. Let me share three personal stories in my professional life that validated this conclusion.

In 1965 in Boston, I attended an ASHP General Practice Institute with the objective of learning all I could about this new and growing pharmacy movement in the United States called hospital pharmacy practice. At the time, I was a newly hired director of pharmacy in a 300-bed hospital in Lubbock, Texas, with no experience beyond two years of disillusioning retail store management. I was sampling this new and different practice with one eye while the other was looking to save enough money to attend medical school as soon as possible. At that weeklong meeting I met and interacted with local and renowned national leaders and hospital pharmacy practitioners such as innovator John Webb who gave us a tour at Massachusetts General Hospital and Joe Oddis, a dynamic young Executive Vice President at ASHP. I was immediately blown away by their enthusiasm and passion for the patient and the profession.

These two men had a professional sense of purpose, a genuine concern for the patient, and an open mind and creative spirit for sharing innovative ways to make drug therapy and patient care safer and more effective. This passionate vision for pharmacy was so far beyond the simple blind filling of drug baskets—the prevalent practice in hospitals at the time. There was an almost electric, exciting, and profound sense of professional brotherhood as we shared common frustrations and challenges with the status quo. This frustration was somehow always balanced with a shared positive belief in a vision of pharmacy practice that can better serve the patient tomorrow than today. Bottom line . . . I was hooked and from then until today, I have embraced this passionate vision for advanced pharmacy practice. I returned to West Texas with a newfound vision—a vision for care that our team grew to translate into a wonderful reality over the next 13 years at our hospital. Our team developed and fully implemented one of the first comprehensive unit-dose and IV admixture systems in the Southwest. The innovative system we created also included a comprehensive pharmacy nurse program responsible for administering medications 24x7 to the patients in the hospital that had ultimately grown to 700 beds.

Fast forward to 1987 where I was nine years into pursuing another such practice vision by building and leading a successful pharmacy system and innovative clinical team at a large integrated health system (Scott & White) in Central Texas. However, the economic realities of the diagnosis-related group (DRG) reimbursement system imposed in the mid-1980s were challenging hospitals' financial resources with budget pressures and staff cuts. Progressive pharmacy practice moved far beyond the walls of traditional central pharmacy to the patient care units, surgery, and intensive care area satellites. Our previously successful leadership model faced the new challenges of a decentralized model of practice, dramatic clinical services expansion into the larger patient care team, and incessant financial pressures. After experiencing remarkable success, we encountered resistance to continued improvement of patient care at every level. After a brief struggle with those realities and flirting with disillusion with our pharmacy vision, we mustered our professional strength and with collective passion took the leadership team offsite for a two-day retreat we called Renaissance '87. At that retreat our team shared frustrations, challenges, and creative solutions while confirming a common commitment to our passionate pharmacy vision for improving care.

Once again the infectious will, ideas, and creative plans for execution came alive within all of us. We returned to our pharmacy with a fresh sense of commitment and a renewed passion shared by an expanded team of fully engaged pharmacy leaders and staff. At least annually after that pivotal experience, the team regularly "retreated" to renew and update that passionate vision. This shared culture of leadership—accountability far beyond any traditional top-down structure I alone could have mustered—carried our expanding pharmacy momentum to new heights and remarkable patient care achievements over the next seven years!

Once again fast forward roughly seven years to 1994 at that same health system. Our pharmacy team continued to pursue our passionate vision for improving care, expanding pharmacy's influence and proven practice approach into the integrated systems' expanding ambulatory care world of clinics, retail pharmacies, and even managed care pharmacy! However, with all that relative success came increasing pressure to justify our rapid growth beyond traditional acute care limitations. My hospital responsibilities expanded and my compensation lagged. I still enjoyed the work with a passion for patient care but felt unappreciated, overworked, and again flirted with professional disillusion. Our clinical efforts were consistently challenged in spite of proven outcomes and return-on-investment economics that exceeded national metrics and any department in our health system. I considered several enticing offers luring me in potential new directions. I personally retreated, took time for self-reflection, and re-examined my beliefs and my state of professional passion. This time I conferred with trusted team members and my now extended national network of pharmacy colleagues.

I ultimately came to the conclusion that it was that same passionate vision for the profession striving to better serve our patients that means the most to me and sustains me. It was not financial compensation, titles, personal recognition or appreciation at any level! From that re-awakening, I finally came to fully understand and realize a true professional actually works for something far greater—that passionate vision and nothing else. This realization frees us to let go of the rest of those concerns and to move on to address the next inevitable challenge! From that moment until fall 2003 when I left that practice after a wonderful 25+ years, this shared passion carried me and our team to new heights of progressive patient care in a fully integrated health care system despite the continuing struggles with budget cuts, politics of working for three corporate bosses, and other threats to progress along the way.

My three personal stories sprinkled across almost four decades of health-system leadership practice demonstrate one clear and sustaining principle that will ensure our professional success: Nurture a shared passion for the patient with the belief and vision that continually improving pharmacy practice will make tomorrow better and safer than today for our patients! This passion is not about the drugs, the systems or processes, recognition or rewards, but rather the people we serve—the patient and family, our pharmacy team, and our expanded patient care team of physicians, nurses, and ancillary support staff—all who share our common passionate vision!

Find this passion for yourself, nurture it with your team, and there will be no limit to your professional success . . . and a fulfilling life!

Sincerely,
*Billy Woodward*

# David A. Zilz

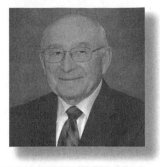

## *The Pharmacist–Physician Relationship: It's about Trust*

Soon after meeting DZ, as he is known to many, it will become clear to you that this is a very proud and passionate person with a wide range of interests. He takes almost as much pride in his commercial driver's license as he does in his pharmacy license. Dave is as passionate about forestry and the environment as he is about pharmacy, health care, and leadership.

Dave spent his entire career in leadership positions at the University of Wisconsin Hospital. Not only was he successful in his roles at the University, he also provided leadership to many other organizations including the University Healthsystem Consortium and the American Society of Health-System Pharmacists. The educational model for training pharmacists for practice and advanced training for leadership is also one of his passions. His strong support of uniting the education mission of the University of Wisconsin School of Pharmacy with the pharmacy practice mission of the University of Wisconsin Hospital Department of Pharmacy has certainly produced skilled practitioners and leaders who have improved the care of patients. Most who know him well would say that his investing in the current and future leaders through mentorship will be one of the cornerstones of his legacy. And as you might imagine, he is a very thoughtful leader.

Dave received his bachelor of science and master of science degrees from the University of Wisconsin. When asked to reflect on his career and wisdom to pass on to current and future pharmacy leaders, his message was clear: *The pharmacist–physician relationship is important, and the relationship is about trust.*

Dear Young Pharmacist,

A physician leader stated to me "We don't need more spectators! If you are here when I am here (seven days a week), are willing to get your hands dirty as I frequently do, and if I can count on you to follow up in a reliable way every time a drug decision is made, we will get along just fine and be a great team." I understood exactly what he needed in a pharmacist partner: you have to be accountable, accessible, and graciously assertive representing all areas of pharmacy practice.

One constant in your career will be a relationship with physicians and the medical community. The relationship is extremely important because almost everything you do in practice or policy development regarding patients' use of medications will require some level of partnership with physicians. You will learn that the pharmacy and medical professions share common values, beliefs, and philosophies of practice in achieving optimum outcomes for the dollars spent on drug therapies. Of course, the emotions of this relationship will span a continuum of frustration during times of disagreement to elation due to great patient care resulting from exceptional teamwork. You bring tremendous value to this relationship, and you own at least 50 percent of the frustration and the elation resulting from the relationship.

In the 1960s, I began my journey of understanding and valuing the pharmacist–physician relationship and its impact on the success of pharmacy practice and services. Winston Durant, our Director of Pharmacy at the University of Wisconsin, believed that pharmacists working directly with physicians in patient care areas to determine the medication needs of patients and managing the medication-use system would improve medication safety and increase nursing efficiency. This was clearly the right model for us. It was also very clear to Mr. Durant that this model's success required an understanding of physicians, their thought processes, and practice to partner with them and fulfill the patients' medication needs. He strongly believed and instilled in many of us that a good pharmacist–physician relationship is an absolute necessity to achieve the optimum use of medications. Since early in my career, my assignments enabled me to work with physicians in all practice settings at all times of the day and night and especially to attend many committee meetings and conferences that enhanced my understanding of their practices.

I learned early in my career that the medication-related systems and processes are important not only to pharmacists, but they are extremely important to physicians' efficiency and productivity. I spent time in rural Wisconsin with a solo practice, primary care physician to understand his practice and determine how pharmacists could help in rural areas. He welcomed my observation of his practice, and to my surprise invited me to stay as a guest in his family's home for two weeks. What a great opportunity! This physician saw as many as 120 patients per day as a solo practitioner. There were numerous evenings when I was awakened by a knock on the bedroom door to accompany him on medical emergencies such as auto accident injuries, the birth of a baby, or an unexpected hospital admission. I witnessed over 1,000 patient encounters. However, the process of documenting medication therapy and communicating with the pharmacies in town was cumbersome. Once he decided on a drug therapy, he carefully documented the therapy in the medical record and often spent significant time on the phone communicating with local pharmacists. After observing these time-consuming activities, I approached pharmacists from the two pharmacies in town and shared my observation. Both pharmacists decided to change the system and process and install "hot lines" that would be answered by pharmacists and would significantly decrease the physician's phone time. Additionally, they would maintain and share their drug therapy documentation with him to decrease his time required to document therapy. Although these changes might seem insignificant in today's world, these changes significantly improved his productivity, and when I met him 45 years later, he remembered vividly the time I spent with him and continued to express his appreciation for my contribution.

An unusual situation gave me the opportunity to develop a relationship with physicians that transformed my thinking when I had administrative responsibility for pharmacy, respiratory therapy, and materials management. I received a call one weekend that the leader of respiratory therapy was hospitalized with a severe myocardial infarction and emminent premature death. I met with the physician leaders of respiratory and pulmonary function services to determine how to continue to manage the services. During these frequent meetings, a unique relationship developed. We gained a greater understanding and appreciation of each other's needs and practices, and we developed a relationship based on trust. This incident made me realize that our values and beliefs were more aligned than I had previously believed.

In my interactions with the medical community (e.g., medical students, senior medical faculty, committees within organizations, chiefs of staff, government agency officials, etc.), I often found myself in a position—as you will in your career—to improve their regard for pharmacists' ability to care for patients. It is important to understand the organization's governance process and how the physicians' intellect and patient care attitudes might translate into policies that impact pharmacy practice. Do not hesitate to focus on the thought leaders and seek information on issues they address as well as their point of view on issues that are important to you. Be a role model in your organization and volunteer early in the process on broad issues of patient care that might not relate directly to you.

Remember, the pharmacist–physician relationship is really about two professionals with unique and fundamentally complementary knowledge about disease processes, and how medications alter those processes. I think today's pharmacists are very comfortable practicing with physicians because of their clinical training and team-based approaches. However, I need to remind you that working together does not always equate to the sustainable trusting relationship you need to lead change. I always went out of my way to develop these relationships with physicians. You should never forget that pharmacy systems and processes impact the day-to-day work and productivity of physicians. Both professionals depend on overlapping systems to complete their work.

As I bring this letter to a close, there are a few additional observations I made during my career and suggestions that might help in your relationship with physicians.

- Physicians value the evidence-based, comprehensive assessment process, and the depth of basic scientific understanding of the pharmacist. It certainly generates trust and confidence when facing sophisticated therapy planning issues. I encourage you to value this partnership and the complementary skill set and avoid competition for therapeutic superiority.

- Know that pharmacists and physicians are on a similar constructive growth curve regarding health care policy. You will find that with time, maturity, and security there will be more collaboration leading to a level of comfort and predictability with your physician colleagues regarding health care policy. Had I been aware of this, many little issues that got in the way would have been viewed differently.

- Engage in open dialogue with physicians to ensure high-quality patient care and the common good.

- Bring organizational-level thinking to your conversations with physicians. All too often my interface with them was to address a conflict or an immediate issue. Once I learned to expand the scope of my conversation, it provided us a different platform for our discussions. When I raised the level of the discussion with the question, "What else do you think I should know that would be good for the organization?," I almost always received a positive, constructive, and instructive response.

- Exude professionalism in all that you do, and practice pharmacy with a big picture in mind that integrates all pharmacy activities.

Best wishes for a great career!

Sincerely,
*Dave—DZ*

# Final Thoughts

here are many books that contain compilations of letters. A quick search on Amazon yields dozens. Ellyn Spragins' book of letters from very accomplished women writing to their younger selves sparked the idea for this book. We all have tough decisions to make in our careers. Wouldn't it be nice, we thought, if young pharmacists could learn from the experiences—both good and bad—of leading pharmacists in our profession? For the three of us, reading the Spragins' book served as a call to action.

After getting the nod from ASHP on the book proposal, we set out to identify pharmacists with unique stories to tell. We sought stories from which a lesson would emerge that might help enhance the career or personal life of a pharmacist along his or her career journey. As a starting point, we brainstormed the messages we would have wanted to hear along our own career journeys: Handling disappointments, blazing a trail in clinical practice, juggling and balancing the needs of family and a demanding career, facing a serious illness, and the many other things that have prompted us to say, "if I had only known then what I know now." We reflected on the memorable and touching stories we were privileged to hear from those who have lived them. In her presidential address in 2010, Diane Ginsburg told the story of her mother's "every patient" advice that had such an impact on her career. She agreed to share that story again in the pages of this book. Ernie Anderson wrote with a great degree of candor and humility about the loss of a job he had loved and to which he had given his all for 17 years. Joyce Generali provides advice on sticking with your priorities and saying no when it is the right thing to do. We all remembered the cancer battle fought by one of the leaders of our profession, Bob Weber, and were moved to tears when we read his heart-wrenching letter about this dark time in his life.

It became clear early in the development of the book that our profession is rife with great stories and great story tellers. Narrowing the list of potential contributors to a number that could feasibly be included in the book was a significant challenge, but the best kind of problem to have when you are writing a book. We struggled with the challenge and finally used a list of priority topics to guide our invitations to the contributors. This group of extraordinary individuals did not disappoint.

It is our hope that you not only enjoyed reading each letter but also found useful pearls of wisdom to apply in your life and career. We are certain, though, that you did not enjoy reading it as much as we have enjoyed working on it. Our work required us to connect with all the contributors by phone as well as by e-mail. Although we all knew the contributors, we did not know some of them well before starting the book, and there were others we had not spoken with in a long time. (Don't lose touch with those who matter . . . .Sage advice we should have included in the book!) We enjoyed reconnecting and hearing their remarkable stories. Friendships have been made and rekindled through the writing of this book, and our lives have been enriched.

The contributors' stories also caused us to reflect on how far our profession has come over the last five decades. We have seen a seismic shift in the education and training of pharmacists and in the roles that pharmacists play in the delivery of health care. Pharmacy has evolved into a critical element of patient care; pharmacists are now part of the essential health care team. Everyone with whom we worked on this book expressed optimism about the current state and the future of our profession. It is our hope that in some small way these contributors' advice will help "grease the skids" to advance the careers of our future pharmacy leaders.

We thank you in advance for the many contributions that you will no doubt make to the patients you serve and to our profession. We wish you all the best on your career journey.